THE COMPLETE GUIDE TO

Adaptogens

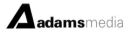

Adams Media
An Imprint of Simon & Schuster, Inc.
57 Littlefield Street
Avon, Massachusetts 02322

First Adams Media hardcover edition July 2018

ADAMS MEDIA and colophon are trademarks of Simon & Schuster.

For information about special discounts for bulk purchases, please contact Simon & Schuster Special Sales at 1-866-506-1949 or business@simonandschuster.com.

The Simon & Schuster Speakers Bureau can bring authors to your live event. For more information or to book an event contact the Simon & Schuster Speakers Bureau at 1-866-248-3049 or visit our website at www.simonspeakers.com.

Interior design by Sylvia McArdle and Colleen Cunningham
Interior photographs by Harper Point Photography
Interior illustrations by Katrina Machado

Manufactured in the United States of America

10 9 8 7 6 5 4 3 2 1

Library of Congress Cataloging-in-Publication Data
Noveille, Agatha, author.
The complete guide to adaptogens / Agatha Noveille.
Avon, Massachusetts: Adams Media, 2018.
Includes bibliographical references and index.
LCCN 2018011469 (print) | LCCN 2018018882 (ebook) | ISBN 9781507207840 (hc) |
ISBN 9781507207857 (ebook)
LCSH: Herbs--Therapeutic use. | Healing. | BISAC: HEALTH & FITNESS / Herbal Medications. | HEALTH & FITNESS / Alternative Therapies. | HEALTH & FITNESS / Healing.
LCC RM666.H33 (ebook) | LCC RM666.H33 N683 2018 (print) | DDC 615.3/21--dc23
LC record available at https://lccn.loc.gov/2018011469

ISBN 978-1-5072-0784-0
ISBN 978-1-5072-0785-7 (ebook)

Contains material adapted from the following title published by Adams Media, an Imprint of Simon & Schuster, Inc.: *Adaptogens* by Agatha Noveille, copyright © 2016, ISBN 978-1-4405-9639-1.

THE COMPLETE GUIDE TO

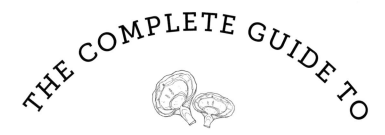

Adaptogens

From **Ashwagandha** to **Rhodiola**,
Medicinal Herbs That
Transform and Heal

AGATHA NOVEILLE

Adams Media
New York   London   Toronto   Sydney   New Delhi

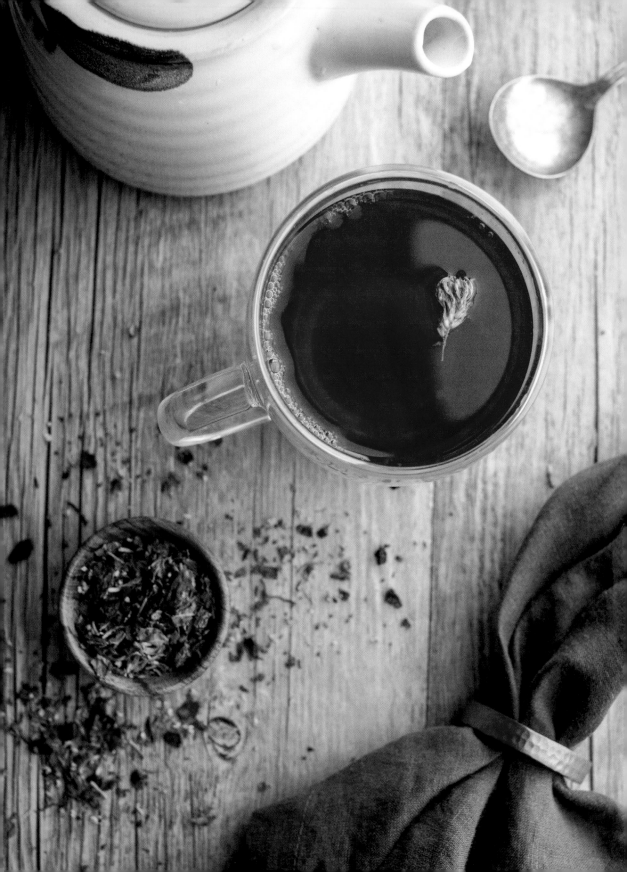

CONTENTS

ADAPTOGENIC RECIPES FOR WELLNESS

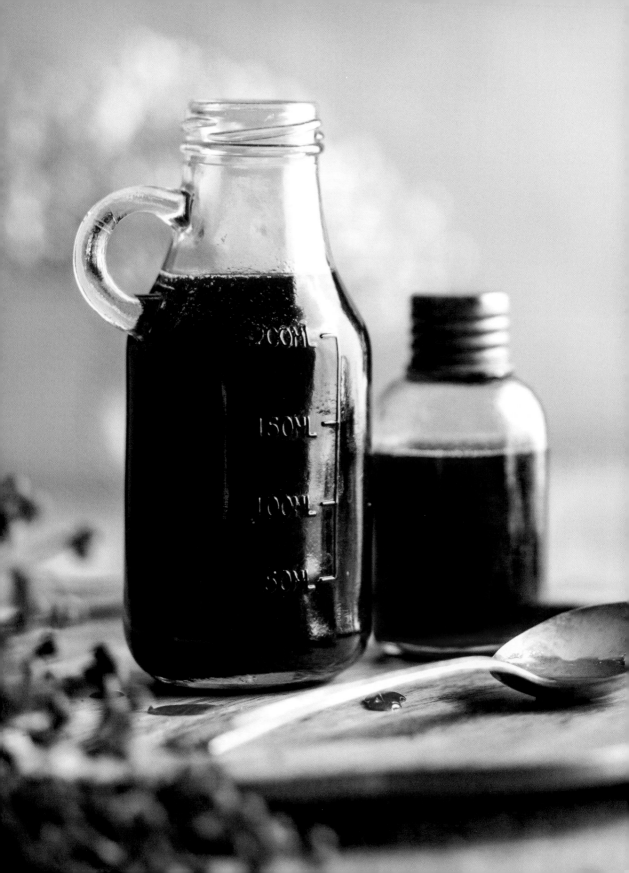

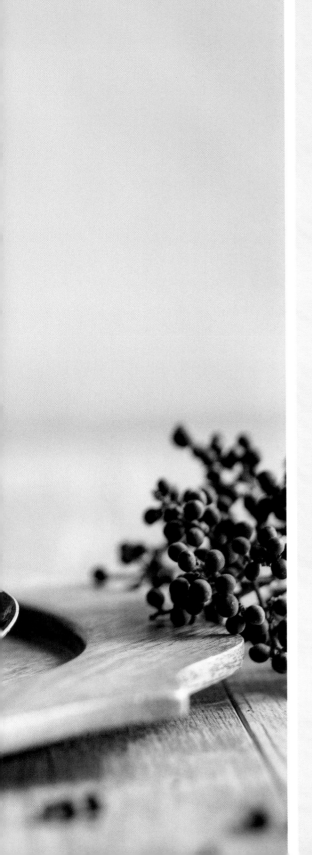

Introduction

The human quest for longevity, youthfulness, and rejuvenation has spanned hundreds of years and taken many forms. From the medieval obsession with alchemy and the elixir of life to the modern fascination with superfoods, it seems that we have always had a drive to do more, be more, and set new standards for health and vitality.

Many years ago, the Soviet Union instructed their scientists to open a new chapter in this quest. They were ordered to search for and develop substances that would allow their athletes, military personnel, and even chess players to excel above and beyond, to have an edge in stamina, strength, endurance, and mental abilities that would bring them international glory. After much work, these scientists focused their research on, of all things, herbs—a very specific group of herbs that became known as adaptogens. American ginseng, eleuthero, rhodiola, and holy basil are just a few examples of the plants that we now know as adaptogens. These remarkable plants have been shown to have a gentle but measurable influence on immunity, sleep, stress levels, energy, and endurance.

Whether you are interested in honing your mental abilities to a razor-sharp level, want to give your athleticism a boost, or are looking for ways to include tonic herbs as part of a healthy lifestyle, adaptogens have so much to offer for everyday well-being.

There are fabulous resources available to teach you about the many traditional uses and modern research regarding these herbs, but this book is different. It shows you how to take these amazing herbs and add them into your daily routines with flair! By making your own extracts, elixirs, and teas, you will save money, have a high-quality product, and end with something that's unique rather than an off-the-shelf item. You can tailor your creations to be exactly what you want or need them to be!

Adaptogens lend themselves well to a variety of creative recipes, and working with them in this way is a pleasure. Rather than another expensive vitamin pill to pop or a bitter-tasting herbal extract to toss back while pinching your nose, you can experiment with tasty teas, yummy syrups, or fun and interesting snacks to incorporate adaptogens into your life.

Adaptogens can become a valuable part of your healthy lifestyle. They are also a great way to begin working with herbs in general. Thanks to their safety (an herb must be nontoxic and safe for extended use to qualify as an adaptogen), they are some of the easiest and most accessible herbs to work with for the average person. With a few general guidelines in place, you can approach these herbs with confidence. Turn the page to find out what you need to get started creating your first DIY adaptogen recipes, and follow in the footsteps of others who have explored some of the most compelling quests in human history: How much can we do? How much can we become? What is the full potential for our health and vitality?

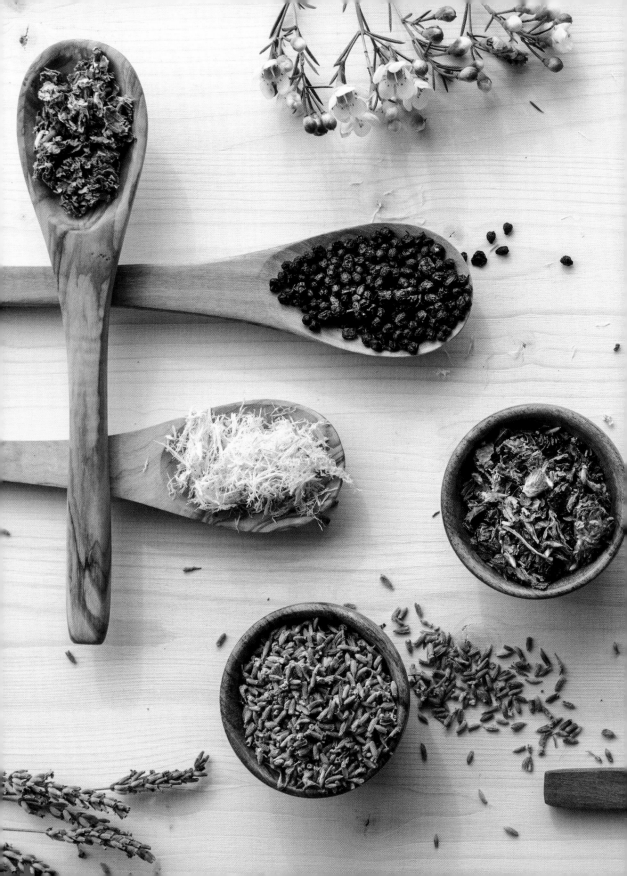

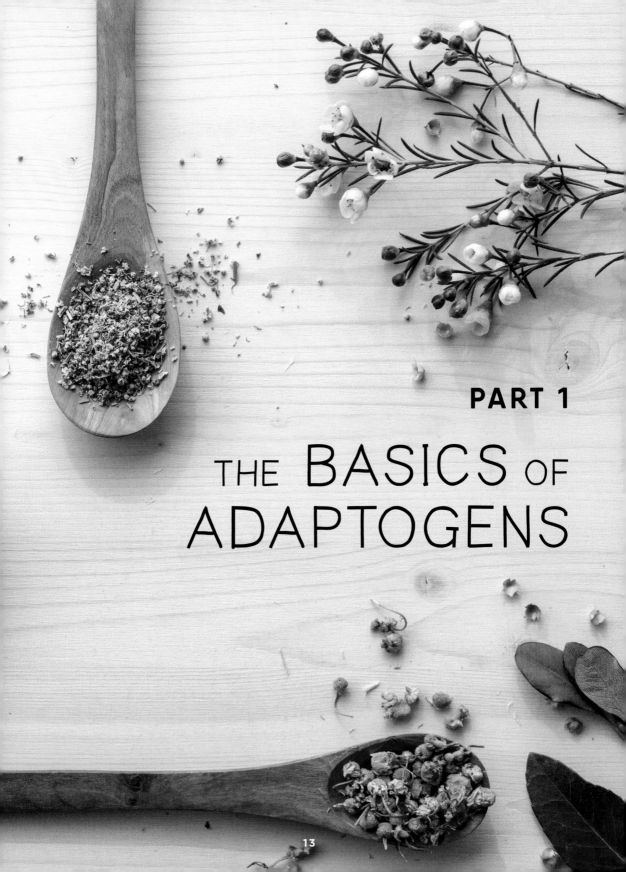

PART 1

THE BASICS OF ADAPTOGENS

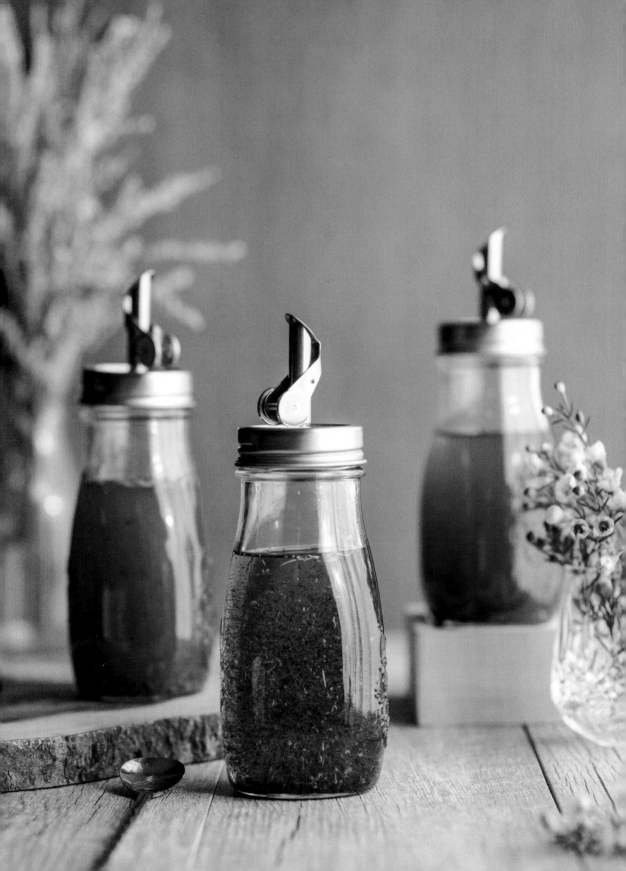

CHAPTER ONE

UNDERSTANDING AND USING ADAPTOGENS

Many people are looking for ways to be healthy that go beyond the vitamin bottle. They are looking for ways to increase vitality that are less about taking a pill and more about making different lifestyle choices, incorporating nutrient-dense foods, and utilizing the basic tenets of many ancient forms of healing, including herbalism, in daily life. During this quest for optimum health and vitality, many people come across the concept of adaptogenic herbs.

What Are Adaptogens?

The concept of plants with revitalizing or restorative properties that can enhance health has been around for thousands of years, although "adaptogen" is a modern word that has only been used to describe them since the 1940s. Many of the herbs that we know as adaptogens today were first used generations ago in Ayurveda (the traditional system of herbalism in India) and in traditional Chinese medicine (TCM).

In Ayurveda, for example, herbs such as amla, shatavari, and holy basil are classified as rasayana herbs. Rasayanas are herbs that increase vitality and are believed to promote youthfulness and increase resistance to illness. In modern herbalism, we use these three herbs along with many other rasayanas as adaptogens.

One of the concepts of traditional Chinese medicine groups herbs into three categories based on their actions and safety of use. Many herbs in the first category, sometimes translated as "superior" herbs, are valued for their tonic and harmonizing influence on overall health. Many herbs that we know as adaptogens today belong to this class of herbs, such as he shou wu, eleuthero, and schisandra.

So how did we come to describe these herbs as adaptogens? In the late 1940s, the government of the then-USSR instructed its scientists to create a substance that could be used to increase the performance of the country's athletes, military personnel, and even elite chess players, so that they could dominate and excel in every international arena.

We owe the modern word "adaptogen" to the Soviet doctor and scientist Nikolai V. Lazarev. In 1947, he created the word from the Latin word *adaptare*, meaning "to adjust." He used it to mean a substance that raises the non-specific resistance of the body to stress so that the body is better able to adapt to stressful circumstances.

Eventually, the Soviet research into adaptogens—which had a strict focus on safety—turned away from chemical substances such as dibazol and began to focus on American ginseng. From there, research branched out to include other plants that also belonged to the Araliaceae family, such as eleuthero, and then to an even broader selection of herbs.

By 1968, Israel I. Brekhman, PhD, and Dr. I.V. Dardymov had developed the functional definition that has evolved into the understanding of adaptogens that we have today. According to the definition used by Brekhman and Dardymov:

1. An adaptogen is nontoxic to the recipient.

2. An adaptogen produces a nonspecific response in the body—an increase in the power of resistance against multiple stressors, including physical, chemical, or biological agents.

3. An adaptogen has a normalizing influence on physiology, irrespective of the direction of change from physiological norms caused by the stressor.

Although this is the first recorded functional definition of adaptogens, there is no "official" definition. But, like this original definition, most modern descriptions include the concepts that adaptogens:

• Are nontoxic

• Increase resistance to multiple stressors

• Help normalize physiological responses despite prior stress-related changes in the body

Consistent Use

A pressing question for many people when they begin using adaptogens is: "Should I take a break from using adaptogens? If so, how often?" Adaptogens actually seem to work better with regular use, and you don't usually need to worry about them putting a particular strain on the body or your body building up a tolerance. Personally, I like choosing one adaptogen to use at least once a day for a few months at a time before switching over to another or taking a rest. I find that it helps to periodically reevaluate my personal health goals and concerns when deciding which adaptogen to use. Our bodies change over time and it makes sense to change our adaptogens to match what's going on with our health.

Safety

Thanks to their unusual influence on the body's ability to handle stress, adaptogens can offer a unique way to support your health. They can offer you a way to support your best possible health and performance, but moderation is key. In other words, they shouldn't be a substitute for good self-care practices, such as getting enough sleep and eating well!

It's true that adaptogens and other herbs are "all natural," but you should still take proper precautions. There is always the possibility of getting too much of a good thing, having an allergic reaction, or experiencing side effects when taking herbs alongside prescription medications. Some of the most important safety considerations are included in the profile for each herb in the glossary section (see Chapter 2), but it's always a good idea to consult with your primary health care provider before including adaptogens in your diet.

Your current state of health and your health history are important considerations when deciding to incorporate any herbs into your diet, and this is especially true of adaptogens. For example, some adaptogens, like licorice, can increase blood pressure in sensitive individuals. Typically, this is only a problem if the licorice is consumed in large amounts for extended periods of time, but if you are prone to high blood pressure, you should use licorice with awareness and only after you speak with your doctor. Another example is holy basil. Although a wonderful adaptogen and nervine (an herb that supports the nervous system), this herb may not be suitable for use during pregnancy.

It becomes doubly important to know safety information on the herbs you work with if you are on prescribed medications. In some cases, herbs can affect your metabolism or alter the way the liver processes medications. Herbs, including adaptogens, may have a synergistic or antagonistic influence when taken with pharmaceuticals. It's best to do some careful research and speak with your doctor or pharmacist before proceeding if you take a daily prescription medication.

Usage Guidelines

By using these guidelines and treating adaptogens with the respect they deserve as potent allies for health, you can incorporate these wonderful herbs into your daily life and enjoy their many benefits.

Watch Serving Sizes

When you add herbs to your diet, it's important to remember that more isn't necessarily better. Each individual herb has a particular safe range that shouldn't be exceeded, and you should be careful not to combine full servings of several herbs that have similar actions. For instance, it's better to take one serving of a formula of herbs that promote a good night's sleep than to take a full serving of four different individual herbs that all promote sleep. Adaptogens are no different. They are safe herbs, but taking too much of one or more at a time or over the course of a day can leave you feeling jittery or aggressive. With prepackaged, off-the-shelf herbal supplements, it's important to follow the recommended serving size and directions that come with the product. Make sure that you know the basic guidelines on correct serving sizes for the preparations you choose to make at home. Be mindful of how many recipes you use and how many herbal supplements with adaptogens in them that you take on any given day, and keep your total servings (including any off-the-shelf supplements that include adaptogens) to three or fewer servings.

For Adults Only

It may be tempting to incorporate adaptogens into the diets of the whole family, but what may be a wonderful herb for an adult may be less desirable for a child. Some adaptogens appear to have a very potent influence on the endocrine system, and may alter hormone levels in adults. Because children are still growing and their endocrine system is developing, the use of adaptogens with preteens and even teens is a very complex subject.

There are a few adaptogens that are exceptions to this rule, but in most cases it would be best to speak with a qualified herbalist about the child's specific situation before making the decision to add adaptogens to his or her diet.

Amber Glass Bottles

Herbalists seem to have a bit of an obsession with brown glass bottles, but there is a reason for it. Brown glass helps keep out the light, which protects the extracts inside and preserves them better. If you do need to keep them in a clear glass canning jar (say, if you run out of empty bottles or you are on a tight budget), be sure to keep the extracts in a cool, dark cupboard when you aren't using them. Personally, I prefer to skip the dropper-top bottles that are popular and use plain screw-top caps instead. I use either a set of measuring spoons or the cap of the bottle when measuring out a serving.

Tools and Supplies

Many of the tools and supplies needed for the recipes and projects in this book are probably already in your kitchen. Check your drawers and cabinets for the following basic tools:

- Glass or enamel pot
- Mixing bowl
- Strainer
- Mixing spoons
- Measuring utensils
- Glass canning jars
- Teakettle
- French press

Glass or Enamel Pot

A medium to large glass or enamel pot with a lid is very useful for making herbal infusions and decoctions, and is generally better to use than metal because it won't leach into or react with your recipes.

Mixing Bowl

Whether blending ingredients to make a tea or creating more elaborate recipes, a large glass mixing bowl is essential.

Strainer

Having a mesh strainer available makes the potentially messy process of filtering herbal infusions, extracts, and oils much easier. A jelly-making cone or bag on a stand is also helpful. Coffee filters often work well in a pinch, but they are prone to tearing, and it's nice to have a stronger, reusable solution available.

Mixing Spoons

If you aren't a fan of wooden spoons, make sure to choose a utensil that is durable, nonreactive, and heat resistant. A silicone spoon or spatula is a good alternative.

Measuring Utensils

Glass has the benefit of being see-through so you can get exact measurements from the side, but stainless steel measuring cups and spoons are also durable and easy to clean.

Glass Canning Jars

Glass canning jars are the perfect vessels for infusing herbal oils, extracts, and elixirs and storing tea and powdered herb blends. Two sizes, 16- and 32-ounce (pint and quart sizes), are the most versatile and will work for most of the projects in this book. The metal bands and lids used for canning are prone to rusting when exposed to the herbal extract and vinegar-making processes, but plastic screw-top lids can be purchased for glass canning jars and are a good alternative.

Teakettle

In a pinch, you can simply heat water in your saucepan, but a teakettle is nice for easy pouring into a cup or French press. Finding a sturdy teakettle can be tough, but it's worth it in the long run to invest in one that will last. If you choose one that has a whistle, look for a hinge that keeps the whistle firmly attached so it doesn't get lost. Enamel teakettles can be beautiful, but they may be prone to chipping, cracking, or other wear and tear on the bottom where they come in direct contact with the stovetop, so treat them with extra care.

French Press

A good French press makes coffee brewing an elegant and simple affair, and a press is just as easily used to make an herbal tea! Why fiddle with other tea-making filters and strainers when a French press serves so admirably? Admittedly, a tea strainer collection can be amusing, especially because they can be found in a wide range of classic to humorous shapes and styles. But for easily making anywhere from a single cup to several at once, or to cut down on the kitchen clutter, a good French press will be perfect.

Stainless Steel

Remember that while glass and enamel mixing bowls and pots are generally best for herbal projects, stainless steel teakettles and French presses are just fine, and have the added benefit of being extra durable and long-lasting. Avoid highly reactive metals like aluminum or copper, since they may alter the taste of or react with herbal ingredients, just as they do in everyday cooking.

Basic Ingredients

Other than herbs, there are a few additional ingredients called for in the recipes. You can pick them up all at once to have on hand, or gather them as you need them for a specific recipe.

Apple Cider Vinegar

Useful for making infused salad dressings, oxymels (a type of syrup made with herbs, vinegar, and honey), and herbal shrubs (drinks made with fruit, sugar, and herbal vinegar), apple cider vinegar is the classic vinegar for the home herbalist. Most people find it more palatable than white vinegar and it also has the benefit of undergoing less processing. A nice extract can be made in many cases using vinegar instead of vodka, which is good for instances when an alcohol-based extract isn't desired. The finished extract will vary some-what from an alcohol-based extract, but is still serviceable.

Vodka and Brandy

Vodka is the easiest ingredient to use for making your own herbal extracts at home. Either an 80 or a 100 proof vodka is just fine, and will yield a 40 percent or 50 percent alcohol extract, respectively. It's widely available and inexpensive. Brandy can make nice extracts as well, and is also used to make elixirs, which generally have the advantage of tasting better than a straight extract. Be sure to keep an eye on the proof of the brandy you select. You will need one that is a minimum of 40 percent alcohol by vol-ume (80 proof) for a good shelf life.

Honey

Honey is used both as a sweetener and as a carrier or preservative in some of the recipes in this book. If you can, get to know a local beekeeper or farm where you can be sure the bees are being well cared for and the honey is sustainably harvested. If not, choose your honey company carefully—commercial beekeeping practices are often less than ideal. If you don't wish to use honey, you can try substituting agave nectar, brown rice syrup, or maple syrup. Be aware that using one of these substitutes may change the consistency of the finished recipe and may shorten its shelf life, but there is no reason you shouldn't experiment if you so desire! I've noted my favorite substitutions for each recipe where I think it might be helpful.

Olive Oil or Sesame Oil

To keep things simple, the recipes in this book all call for olive oil regardless of whether the recipe is topical or edible in nature. I find that olive oil holds up admirably well for both purposes and is as stable during a heat-infusing method for topical oils as it is for cooking. Extra-virgin olive oil has a more noticeable flavor than virgin olive oil, but either one may be used.

Basic Skills

If you can find your way around the kitchen without too much trouble, you will have no problem navigating most of the recipes in this book. In fact, if you have ever brewed a cup of tea, then you are familiar with the process of making infusions and decoctions. These are the two most basic herbal preparations, made with nothing more than hot water and plant material, and they can be taken internally or applied externally as a wash or added to a bath.

Infusions are herbal preparations made with leaves and flowers, and are made almost exactly the same way as brewing a cup of tea. The herbal leaves or flowers (usually 1–2 teaspoons per 8 ounces of water) are added to a cup of hot water and allowed to steep. The main difference between an infusion and making a regular cup of tea is the length of time the herbs are allowed to steep. Whereas a beverage tea like green tea is usually only steeped for 3 minutes, or 5 at most, herbal infusions are best if allowed to steep for at least 10 minutes.

Decoctions are made by simmering tougher herbal materials like roots, barks, and dried berries for 10–20 minutes and then allowing the herbs to steep. The simmering process breaks down and softens the tough cellulose of the plant's cell walls so that the beneficial compounds are released into the water.

There is one skill that you might not be familiar with, though: how to make an herbal extract, sometimes called a tincture. You may be familiar with extracts from the little amber dropper bottles of liquid herbs on the shelf at your local health food store or herb shop. For most of the herbal recipes in this book, you can either use a store-bought extract or make your own extract at home.

Alcohol-based extracts are some of the most efficient herbal preparations to make and they have a good shelf life. Made and stored correctly, an alcohol-based extract can last up to ten years. The most common way to make an extract is to allow fresh or dried herbs to steep in a mixture of alcohol and water for a minimum of two weeks in a process called maceration. A 40 percent alcohol-by-volume solution is usually perfect for dried materials, so an 80 proof vodka works well because it is inexpensive and readily available. The most common ratio of herbs to alcohol with this process is 1:5. A "folk" method can also be used for most herbs: simply place the herbal material into a glass canning jar and add enough vodka to cover.

For the more scientifically minded, the recipe to remember when making a 1:5 extract is:

> *1 part ground herb by weight (usually given in grams)*
> *+ 5 parts vodka by volume (usually given in milliliters)*

If you are used to ounces, the same ratio still applies, but you will be working with two types of ounces: ounces by weight for the first measurement and ounces by volume for the second.

Yields will vary a little depending on the herbs—some herbs will absorb more of the vodka and be harder to press out, but you can usually expect at least an 80 percent yield. Of course, you can adjust your numbers up or down to make larger or smaller batches of extract, but 4 ounces is a great place to start. It fits nicely in a quart-sized canning jar, and will usually last about a month if you are using it three times a day.

Here's how to make a basic extract with the most common method. It will take around two weeks of maceration before it is ready for use.

PROJECT
Make an Herbal Extract by Maceration

For best results, use herbs that have been powdered. The more finely the herb is broken down, the easier it is for the vodka to go to work softening and extracting the plant material. A coffee grinder can be a good tool for powdering a cut and sifted herb.

YIELDS APPROXIMATELY 4–5 OUNCES

INGREDIENTS

1 ounce by weight (or 29g) dried, powdered herb of your choice
5 ounces by volume (or 145ml) vodka

How to Make

1   Use a quart-sized canning jar, making sure it is clean and dry. Place the measured herb into the jar, then pour in the vodka.

2   Place the lid on the jar and gently shake the herbs and vodka until they are combined. Check the level of alcohol in your jar daily for 2 weeks, and give it a gentle shake each day. Different herbs will absorb different quantities of vodka, so you may need to add a little extra at some point so that there is always enough to cover the herbs.

3   At the end of 2 weeks, allow the jar of extract to rest for a day so that all of the herbal material sinks to the bottom of the jar. Place a colander or strainer over a large bowl and line the colander with a piece of clean muslin cloth. Gently pour the extract through the cloth-lined colander. Next, spoon the slurry from the bottom of the jar into the middle of the cloth, and gather the edges of the cloth together to make a bundle. Twist the bundle to squeeze out as much of the leftover extract as possible.

4   Compost the herbal material in the bundle, and wash and dry the cloth to use again later. Pour the finished extract into a clean amber glass bottle. Label the bottle with the name of the extract and the date it was pressed.

How to Make an Extract by Percolation

If you follow the previous basic extract-making process, you will need to wait a minimum of two weeks before your extract is ready to press. But maceration isn't the only way to make an extract. The same process of percolation that you may know from brewing your morning coffee can be used to make a batch of extract in a single afternoon. Percolation extraction for herbs was first described in *Remington's Pharmaceutical Sciences*, originally published in the 1880s, and was popularized for modern herbalists by James Green and the late Michael Moore.

To make an extract by percolation, finely ground herbs are moistened with alcohol, then packed into a glass funnel made from the neck of a repurposed bottle. The amount of alcohol needed for the extract is then poured into the funnel and allowed to drip down through the powdered herbs. The drip speed is regulated by tightening or loosening the cap on the end of the funnel. Instructions for making your own percolation funnel can be found later in this chapter.

For a 1:5 percolation extract, you will use the same amounts of herbs and vodka as you do for a maceration extract, but you will also need some extra vodka to moisten the plant material when you first begin. Also, although you can use cut and sifted herbs for a normal extract, you must use powdered herbs for an extract made by percolation.

As you begin, it helps to remember that packing the funnel is a bit of an art, and may take some trial and error. The first layer will be the most loosely packed, and the final layer will be the most densely packed. The reason for this is to allow the vodka to flow steadily and smoothly through the herb.

The process is divided up into three stages to make it easier to follow. Although it may seem like a lot of steps to follow, once you have made an extract this way a few times it will go very quickly and easily. Here are the tools you will need in order to make a percolation extract:

Tools

- Glass mixing bowl

- Glass measuring cup (optional)

- Homemade glass funnel

- 2 coffee filters

- Chopstick

- Wooden dowel

- Weight small enough to fit in the widest part of the funnel, such as a clean, flat stone or a few flattened glass marbles

- Quart-sized glass canning jar

Make an Herbal Extract by Percolation

YIELDS APPROXIMATELY 4–5 OUNCES

INGREDIENTS

1 ounce by weight (or 29g) dried, powdered herb of your choice
5 ounces by volume (or 145ml) vodka
Extra vodka as needed

Stage One: Packing the Glass Funnel

This stage is the basic setup for making a percolation extract. You will moisten the herbal material so that it softens, and then pack it into the glass funnel.

1 Pour the finely powdered herb you will be using into a glass mixing bowl. Stir in a little vodka at a time, until the herb is evenly moist. It should be damp enough to easily pack into the funnel in the following steps. Avoid making a messy, soupy slurry—go for "making a sandcastle" damp. If you like, you can be more technical about this: pack the dry powdered herb into a glass measuring cup to get the volume measurement of the powder. Determine $2/3$ of the volume of the herb. That number is the amount of vodka to use. Double-check once you have added all the vodka to make sure all of the herb is moistened, and add a little extra if needed.

2 Trace circles onto two coffee filters using the big opening of your glass funnel. Cut them out and set one aside. Take the other and fold it to make a half circle, then in half again to make a quarter circle.

3 Tease open the center of the folded coffee filter to make a cone.

4 Make sure the cap is securely on the glass funnel. Lightly pack some of the moistened herb into the cone, and slide the packed cone into the neck of the glass funnel. You may need the chopstick to help get it into position, or you may be able to use your fingers.

5   Separate the remaining herb into three portions.

6   Carefully add $\frac{1}{3}$ of the remaining herb to the glass funnel and tamp it down gently using the wooden dowel, focusing on making it level on top. Add the second portion and tamp it down more tightly than the first layer. Add the third portion and tamp it down even more densely than the first and second layers.

Stage Two: Allow the Herb to Rest

Once you have packed the glass funnel, it's time to add the vodka, seal the open end of the funnel, and allow the vodka and herb to rest overnight.

1   Position the second coffee filter circle on top of the tamped down herb, and add the weight on top of the filter.

2   Remove the cap from the glass funnel so that air can escape.

3   Set the packed funnel into the mouth of the large glass canning jar, making sure to position the funnel upright.

4   Add the 5 ounces of vodka slowly and gently to cover the herb. You want the vodka to disturb the packed herb as little as possible. If the funnel was packed properly, the vodka will slowly saturate the powder and begin to drip out of the bottom.

5   It may take a few minutes for the vodka to soak down through the herb and begin to drip. Once the vodka begins to drip steadily from the mouth of the funnel, keep the funnel straight up and down as you lift it out of the jar and screw on the cap, then place the funnel back onto the jar. You should have at least an inch of vodka sitting on top of the powdered herb, probably more.

6   Cover the open end of the glass funnel with a piece of plastic wrap or a zip-top plastic bag to keep the vodka clean. Allow the glass funnel to sit undisturbed overnight.

Stage Three: Percolation

After the herbal material has rested overnight, it's time to adjust the cap to allow the extract to flow through a drop at a time. You should aim for a drop every 1–3 seconds.

1   Remove the plastic to prevent creating a vacuum.

2   Carefully lift the glass funnel straight up and loosen the cap a little at a time until a drop forms every 1–3 seconds. The cap will not need to be loosened much to allow drops to escape, so be careful not to loosen it so much that it falls off.

3   Set the glass funnel back into the jar and allow the extract to percolate into the bottom of the jar over the next few hours.

4   Keep an eye on your extract to make sure there is always space between the cap and the extract below, so that it is dripping freely. Avoid letting the cap become submerged. If you start to run out of space, you can lift the glass funnel gently during percolation and transfer it to an empty canning jar to finish percolating.

5   Your extract should be finished percolating in a few hours. Your time will vary a little depending on how tightly it was packed, what the drip rate is, and even which herb is being used. Transfer your finished extract to a clean amber glass bottle, and label with the date and name of the herb used.

6   There is usually little or no liquid left in the herbs once the extract is finished. The herbs will still appear to be somewhat damp, but all of the good extract is already in the jar below. The leftover herbal material can be composted. There will be very little vodka remaining in the herbs, so it is safe to put them directly into the compost.

Make a Glass Funnel for Percolation Tinctures

To make an extract percolation setup, you will need a glass bottle with a neck, like a wine bottle or the kind used for some brands of sparkling water, and a screw top that fits the bottle. If you can't find a brand of beverage with a screw top at your local bottle shop, you should be able to find an empty one through an online supplier without too much trouble. Companies that sell supplies for home brew enthusiasts are excellent resources.

You will also need a way to score and separate the bottle into two halves. There are many ways that you could go about this. The tutorials that come with bottle-cutting kits and the DIY instructions that you can find by doing a search on *YouTube* will include a method of scoring the glass and sources of alternating heat and cold. Some tutorials will tell you to use things like a candle or burning string for the heat and ice or ice-cold water baths for the other end of the temperature spectrum. Each method will have different levels of success and drawbacks, and some are much more complicated than others.

For simplicity and ease of use, a glass bottle–cutting kit is the best way to go, and that is the method outlined here. Despite the initial expense of purchasing the kit, this method has the advantage of putting the least amount of stress on the glass and providing a clean cut that is easily cleaned up with a little sanding. The kit can always be used later on to make other great DIY projects from recycled glass bottles, so if you enjoy DIY projects in general it's a useful tool to have on hand.

Some kits also come with silicone separation bands. These not only lessen the amount of stress on the glass, which means there is less likelihood of jagged edges or broken bottles, but they also make it a simple matter to separate your bottles with boiling water and cool water only—much less hassle than candles and blow torches. It's up to you which type of kit you choose, but again, the following directions use the easiest method: hot and cold water.

Tools

- Glass bottle–cutting kit

- Safety goggles

- Safety gloves

- Disposable paper safety mask

- Teakettle

- Folded dish towel

Prep Your Bottle

If you've purchased a bottle through a home brew supply company, you can probably skip this step. If you are recycling a beer or wine bottle, wash and dry your bottle thoroughly, and remove all labels and adhesive from the outside of the bottle before you do anything else.

Score the Glass

Once the bottle is clean and the label has been removed, it is time to score the glass. Scoring the glass makes an initial, controlled cut around the circumference of the bottle that will encourage the bottle to break into two clean halves. Fit the bottle-cutting tool from your kit onto the bottle so that the score will be about halfway down the body of the bottle, and follow the directions that came with your kit to make the score. Be sure to wear your safety goggles and gloves.

Apply Heat and Cold

Remove the cutting tool once your bottle has been scored. If your kit came with silicone separation bands, apply them to either side of your score. Heat a kettle of water until it boils. Once the hot water is ready, turn on your kitchen faucet so that it is running a medium stream of cool water. The water does not need to be icy, just cool enough to bring the bottle back down to just below room temperature after the hot water has been applied. Alternating hot and cold water is the process that stresses the score.

Place the folded dish towel into the bottom of the sink so that the bottle won't shatter on the sink when it breaks apart. Hold your bottle in the sink over the towel, and dribble hot water from the kettle over the score. After about 15 seconds, set the kettle aside and place the bottle under the cool water running from your tap. Alternate between hot and cold water as many times as necessary. After a few minutes, half of the bottle will pop off and drop into the sink onto the towel.

Sanding the Edges

If everything goes well, you will have a straight-line cut without jagged edges that need grinding down. Use the sandpaper from your kit, or use a fine-grit silicon carbide sandpaper. The most important thing to remember about sanding glass is that you absolutely must use running water and keep the glass wet while you sand. This is because glass dust is dangerous to inhale. If you want to take extra precautions, you can wear a disposable paper safety mask during this step.

While working over the sink with cool running water, use your sandpaper to round and smooth the edges of your funnel. You can either recycle the bottom of the bottle, or save it for other DIY projects.

Now that you have a handle on the basic tools and techniques, it's time to take a look at the adaptogens themselves.

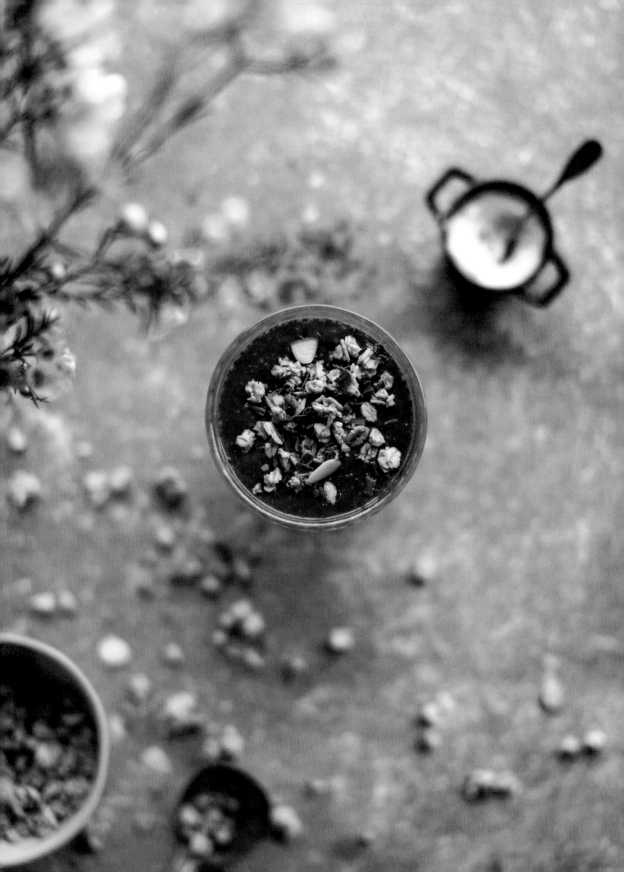

CHAPTER TWO

ADAPTOGENS GLOSSARY

Adaptogenic herbs can be found in every major herbal tradition around the world and grow in a wide range of climates and environments. Although they work broadly across many body systems as a class, each individual adaptogen has nuances behind its actions and areas where it really seems to shine. Knowing some of the background on each adaptogen helps when choosing the best herb for a particular situation, and also provides context from traditional culture, history, and customs that brings the herbs to life in daily use.

Albizia

Albizia julibrissin

Also known as mimosa and silk tree, albizia was introduced as a garden ornamental in the United States and can be found growing wild in many places, because it readily adapted to the climate and naturalized. The pink tasseled flowers and unique leaf shape are easy to identify.

David Hoffmann lists albizia as an adaptogen in his book *Medical Herbalism*.

In traditional Chinese medicine, both the bark and the flowers are used. As nervines, the bark is believed to have a stronger, more grounding effect while the flowers are more uplifting, but they are both used to assist with stress and anxiety.

Albizia is traditionally used for treating diarrhea, insomnia, and poor memory. The bark is also highly valued as herbal support while recovering from injury and physical trauma.

- **USDA Plant Hardiness Zone(s):** 6–9

- **Properties:** analgesic, sedative, nervine relaxant

- **Safety:** Albizia should not be used during pregnancy.

- **Serving Size:** The most common way to use albizia is as an extract. A typical serving of albizia extract is 30–60 drops, and may be taken up to 3 times per day.

Amla

Emblica officinalis syn. *Phyllanthus emblica*

Amla, sometimes known as amalaki, is a popular Ayurvedic tonic from India. Another common name for this herb is Indian gooseberry, although it isn't related to European gooseberry (*Ribes grossularia*). Amla is a medium-sized tree, growing up to 60 feet tall in some cases, and is native to India, southern China, Sri Lanka, Myanmar, and Malaysia. This adaptogen is very sensitive to cold and can only be grown out of doors in USDA zones 9b and warmer.

In Ayurveda, amla fruit is classified as a rasayana and is believed to prolong youthfulness, life, and good memory. Although considered one of the milder adaptogens, this herb nonetheless has a reputation for increasing resistance to disease and nourishing the blood. It is considered an especially effective tonic for restoring the appetite, supporting liver health, and supporting the health of the bones, teeth, and hair. Modern research has shown the fruit to be very rich in vitamin C and antioxidants. The high levels of antioxidants mean that it can play a role in supporting the health of connective tissue, blood vessels, and eyes and help support a healthy inflammatory response. Amla fruit is a key ingredient in the Ayurvedic tonic blends triphala and chyawanprash.

- **USDA Plant Hardiness Zone(s):** 9b–11

- **Properties:** anti-inflammatory, antioxidant, antiviral, mild laxative

- **Safety:** It may be best to space the use of amla and iron, or amla and medications, by 4 hours, because tannins found in amla could potentially interfere with iron absorption or the effectiveness of prescriptions, especially alkaloid medications.

- **Serving Size:** 60–90 drops of 1:4 or 1:5 extract. Use $\frac{1}{2}$–1 teaspoon of amla fruit to 8 ounces of water to make a decoction. Amla can be taken up to 3 times a day.

Ashwagandha

Withania somnifera

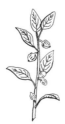

Ashwagandha is an adaptogen that has a reputation as a soothing nerv- ine, and as such it can be well suited for someone who doesn't want or need a stimulating adaptogen. Nervous system health challenges such as anxiety, fatigue, and insomnia from stress are all good reasons to consider ashwagandha.

This adaptogen appears to enhance endocrine function, and can help sup- port an underactive thyroid and support balanced functioning for the tes- tes and adrenal glands. It is often used in Ayurvedic formulas to support fertility and vitality in men.

Ashwagandha has uses as a women's herb, as well. It can be supportive during heavy periods because it is rich in iron, and has been used in Africa as a uterine tonic for women who repeatedly miscarry.

Of course, this adaptogen also has potential uses for supporting the immune system. Ashwagandha has a balancing action and can be used in the presence of either hyper- or hypo-immune function.

A perennial in USDA zone 8 or warmer, ashwagandha can be grown as an annual in cooler climates. The key is to start your ashwagandha seedlings indoors, the same as tomatoes. Ashwagandha needs around 200 days to reach full maturity, but roots that have had at least 100 days may have developed enough for harvest. This herb prefers full sun and alkaline soil.

- **USDA Plant Hardiness Zone(s):** 8–11

- **Properties:** immune tonic, fertility tonic, nervine relaxant, antispasmodic

- **Safety:** This adaptogen is part of the nightshade family, so if you have allergies to plants in this family you may want to consider other adaptogens. Ashwagandha can stimulate the thyroid gland, so it is not ideal for people who have problems with their thyroid being too active. It's also very high in iron, so may not be a good choice if you have a medical condition with excess iron. Ashwagandha is one adaptogen that does have a tradition of use in children, specifically for malnourishment. Although sometimes used as a fertility tonic, this herb may not be suitable for use during pregnancy.

- **Serving Size:** Ashwagandha extracts typically have a serving size in the range of 30–40 drops, up to 3 servings a day. For making a decoction, $\frac{1}{2}$ teaspoon of herb is used in 8 ounces of water, and 2–3 cups can be taken a day.

Astragalus

Astragalus membranaceus

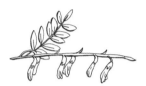

Astragalus is a mild adaptogen and a very good immune system tonic. *Huang Qi*, the Chinese name for astragalus, means "the yellow leader," and refers to the yellow color of the fresh roots as well as the herb's respected place as a premier tonic herb in TCM. Other uses for astragalus include protecting the liver and kidneys from damage caused by viruses or medication, lowering blood sugar, and improving blood flow to the heart.

A perennial herb native to China, Mongolia, Korea, and Siberia, astragalus can be grown in a sunny, sandy spot in gardens in USDA zones 6–11. Astragalus is a member of the legume family, and can grow up to 36" tall. Roots should be harvested from plants that have had time to mature—three- to four-year-old plants are usually good candidates.

- **USDA Plant Hardiness Zone(s):** 6–11

- **Properties:** heart tonic, liver protectant, immune tonic, lung tonic

- **Safety:** Astragalus was traditionally avoided during acute illness because of the belief that it could potentially make the fever last longer or grow stronger, so it may be best to avoid using it if you are feeling under the weather. This is one adaptogen that is widely believed to be safe for children.

- **Serving Size:** 40–80 drops of extract may be used up to 3 times a day. To prepare a decoction of astragalus, use 2 teaspoons of dried herb in 8 ounces of water.

Burdock

Arctium lappa

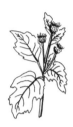

Although there is nothing particularly exotic about burdock, it definitely is worth mentioning alongside some of the other more unusual adaptogens. Although it is more often listed as an alterative than an adaptogen, some herbalists (including Lise Wolff and Christopher Hobbs) do consider it appropriate under both categories.

Burdock is a biennial with weedy growing habits that adapts easily to most growing conditions. If you choose to grow it, you might wish to harvest all of it before it blooms and sets seed, or at least put a brown paper bag over the mature seeds to collect them before they disperse. If you don't, you may find that you won't be able to get rid of it, and may wish you hadn't planted it in the first place! Some varieties of burdock can reach enormous sizes. Most will have small roots ready for harvest after three or four months.

Research has indicated that burdock may protect against mutagenicity (changes in DNA) and have antitumor activity. Herbalists regularly use burdock for poor glandular functions in many areas of the body, including the lymphatic system, the pancreas, the endocrine system, the prostate, the liver, and the spleen. It is also a beneficial adaptogen during recovery from lengthy illnesses and to help restore the body to a state of health.

- **USDA Plant Hardiness Zone(s):** 3–7

- **Properties:** alterative, diuretic, lymphatic and liver tonic

- **Safety:** If you have allergies to plants in the Asteraceae family (such as species of ragweed or wormwood), there is a chance you might have an allergic reaction to burdock. Otherwise, burdock is generally considered a very gentle, safe botanical. Burdock is safe enough that it is even used as a root vegetable.

- **Serving Size:** The serving size for burdock root extract is generally 30–60 drops, up to 3 times a day. For the root, a decoction can be made with as little as a teaspoon or as much as a tablespoon of the dried root.

Cordyceps

Cordyceps sinensis

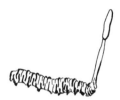

Although most mushrooms are a familiar sight on trees or fallen logs, cordyceps mushrooms are a type of fungus that colonizes caterpillars. After infecting and consuming the larvae of a ghost moth, the fungus fruits and makes a mushroom to release spores. This mushroom, and what's left of the caterpillar, are collected and dried for use as cordyceps.

This particular adaptogen only appears to have been in use in TCM since the 1700s, so it's a relative newcomer. It is somewhat rare in the wild, so it was originally reserved for the emperor and the royal family. Poaching and environmental concerns are a problem thanks to the increased popularity of this herb, but several companies now produce excellent cultivated cordyceps grown on soy instead of caterpillars.

Traditionally used in TCM to support the health of the kidneys and the many concepts believed to be affected by kidney health, cordyceps are used in TCM for infertility, sexual dysfunction, frequent urination, night sweats, dizziness, ringing in the ears, and fatigue. More modern applications include use for athletic performance, as an immune amphoteric, and as a kidney and lung tonic.

- **USDA Plant Hardiness Zone(s):** N/A

- **Properties:** liver and kidney protectant, immune amphoteric, fertility tonic

- **Safety:** Cordyceps is an example of an adaptogen that's great within traditional parameters, but if you overdo it you might experience anxiety, water retention, or a weakened immune system. There is a potential for it to interact with immunosuppressive medications. Cultivated cordyceps may be safer than wild harvested as well as less expensive. After all, in its natural habitat cordyceps grows on a decomposing caterpillar in the presence of potential contaminants such as mold and bacteria.

- **Serving Size:** In an extract form, 20–40 drops of cordyceps can be taken up to 3 times a day. Use $\frac{1}{4}$–$\frac{1}{2}$ teaspoon to make a decoction, and drink only 1–2 cups per day.

Dang Shen

Codonopsis pilosula

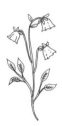

Dang shen is a beautiful flowering vine that is native to China. As a garden plant, it is happiest on a trellis in part shade, with moist, well-drained soil. Dang shen prefers cooler climates, but is sensitive to frost and hardy to USDA zone 6.

The first recorded use of this adaptogen comes from 1670, and can be found in Zhang Lu's *Origin of the Classic Materia Medica*. In TCM, it was often used as a less expensive and milder alternative to ginseng. It has a reputation for improving the digestion and building the blood, and as an immune tonic. Dang shen is also often used in TCM protocols to help support the immune system and lessen side effects during cancer treatments. This adaptogen may also promote healthy blood sugar levels as a hypoglycemic agent, and is beneficial as a digestive system and lung tonic. Dang shen is also known as *codonopsis*.

- **USDA Plant Hardiness Zone(s):** 4–11

- **Properties:** gastroprotectant, hypoglycemic, immune tonic

- **Safety:** Dang shen may be a better option than ginseng for people who find that ginseng is too strong for them. Dang shen can increase hemoglobin counts, so if you have excessive iron levels, this herb may not be a good match for you. Like astragalus, this adaptogen is traditionally avoided during acute illnesses such as colds and flu.

- **Serving Size:** When taking dang shen, 40–80 drops of extract is considered one serving, and can be taken 3 times a day. As a decoction, 1–2 teaspoons of root are used in 8 ounces of water to make one serving, and up to 2 cups of this may be ingested per day.

Eleuthero

Eleutherococcus senticosus

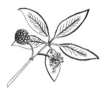

Eleuthero is an understory shrub that can be grown in USDA zones 3–8. It prefers some shade and is adaptable to several different soil conditions. In its native habitat of northern China, it grows in the mountains. Sometimes this herb is mistakenly called Siberian ginseng, even though it is not a true ginseng, because it has properties similar to ginseng. Eleuthero was originally marketed as Siberian ginseng; however, it is now illegal to sell eleuthero as Siberian ginseng in the United State because the name "ginseng" is reserved for *Panax quinquefolius*.

Equally suitable for men and women and especially beneficial for the elderly, eleuthero is gentle, supportive, and good for long-term use. It has nervine actions and offers cognitive support, aids the health of the immune system, and can support healthy cholesterol levels and heart health during stressful times. In addition to being a good everyday adaptogen, eleuthero is an excellent adaptogen for athletes because it supports endurance, shortens recovery times, and appears to protect the immune system during hard training.

This herb is great for those in highly stressful jobs, or who work long hours or have erratic schedules. It often appears to support the quality of sleep while reducing nighttime waking, but doesn't cause drowsiness during the day. Eleuthero may also help to lower blood sugar levels.

For immunity, eleuthero supports the immune system to help reduce incidence of colds and acute illness, but is equally beneficial during recovery from chronic illnesses and surgery.

- **USDA Plant Hardiness Zone(s):** 3-8

- **Properties:** immune tonic, nervine, hypoglycemic, endurance booster

- **Safety:** Eleuthero may react with heart medications and can enhance the effectiveness of macrolide antibiotics and some other medications, so caution should be used when combining eleuthero with prescription drugs.

- **Serving Size:** A serving size of eleuthero is usually 50–100 drops, 3 times a day, or $\frac{1}{2}$–1 teaspoon of dried herb per 8 ounces of water to make a standard decoction.

Ginseng, American

Panax quinquefolius

American ginseng is perhaps one of the best known of the adaptogen herbs. It was, and still is, used by many Native American nations, and thanks to exporting that began in the 1700s has become extremely popular in Chinese herbal medicine as well—often eclipsing Asian ginseng in use and demand.

The two most popular uses for American ginseng are for enhancing energy levels and male libido, but that presents an extremely limited and simplistic view of this herb. Herbalists use it as an immune amphoteric and to support the endocrine system. Other traditional uses include help for dry, chronic coughs; asthma; diabetes; and as a digestive aid. Even though it is one of the most popularized adaptogens, it's one of the most likely to be overly stimulating, and may cause side effects such as headaches, upset stomach, insomnia, anxiety, or high blood pressure.

Unfortunately, the sensationalized status of ginseng has taken a toll on woodland habitats throughout this herb's growing range. When I was a small child, my grandparents retired to a beautiful 60-acre property in the Appalachian Mountains of northeastern Georgia. Both master gardeners, they immediately explored the woods around their new home and found beautiful stands of many different woodland herbs, including American ginseng. Unfortunately, after that first year they never saw it again. The hillside was stripped bare by poachers, and the local ecosystem never recovered in the twenty years they lived there.

Over the last several years, the plight of American ginseng has become even more urgent, but thankfully conservation efforts are underway. American ginseng plants are available through native plant nurseries, and because of the scarcity and the pressure placed on wild populations, farmers and stewards of private forests have begun to produce wild simulated ginseng, also known as certified forest-grown ginseng, for the herbal trade.

Ginseng likes mixed hardwood forests, doesn't tolerate drought or excessively wet conditions, and needs plenty of shade. If you have a suitable growing habitat for ginseng and want to grow your own, you will need lots of patience if your goal is to harvest homegrown roots. Growing ginseng is a lengthy process that requires years for the plant to reach full maturity. This herb can live for a very long time, and the older the plants are, the more valuable the roots. Growers of wild stimulated ginseng will often allow a crop to grow for a minimum of ten years before making a harvest, and some states legally require that ginseng plants be at least five years of age before harvest.

- **USDA Plant Hardiness Zone(s):** 3–8

- **Properties:** central nervous system stimulant, immune tonic, bitter tonic, hypoglycemic

- **Safety:** American ginseng may be too stimulating for some individuals, and may interact with prescription blood thinners.

- **Serving Size:** A serving size of American ginseng extract is generally in the range of 60–100 drops, 3 times per day. To make a tea, 1–2 teaspoons of herb can be used per 8 ounces of water. If you are interested in trying American ginseng but are concerned that a normal serving size may be too strong for you, you can try a half dose and work up to a standard serving.

Ginseng, Asian

Panax ginseng

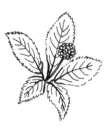

Asian ginseng is one of the most popular tonic herbs in Chinese medicine, and there is a great deal of scientific research that has been done exploring the traditional uses of this herb. Still, in light of the typical Western lifestyle and temperament, it may be one of the least appropriate adaptogens for the average American! It's one of the most stimulating of the adaptogens, which can be a good thing for extremely worn-out or exhausted people who are also addressing lifestyle and diet to support healthy energy levels. However, healthier individuals, especially those who are driven, extremely busy, and fueled by caffeine, may find that it is a bit much. Like other adaptogens, ginseng has an influence on immunity and the adrenals, and may also help protect heart health thanks to high antioxidant levels.

Asian ginseng is also a poster child for what could happen to American ginseng if demand continues to outstrip conservation efforts. Asian ginseng is almost extinct in the wild of its native habitats in Korea and northern China.

- **USDA Plant Hardiness Zone(s):** 3–8

- **Properties:** immune system tonic, adrenal tonic; may help reduce blood sugar levels and protect heart health

- **Safety:** Asian ginseng may increase the effects of blood thinners and medications that lower blood sugar, and could interfere with some types of antidepressants. If you experience headaches, anxiety, high blood pressure, insomnia, or diarrhea while taking Asian ginseng, you may want to try a less stimulating adaptogen or decrease the amount of ginseng you are taking. Avoid drinking caffeine while using ginseng to lessen the chance of negative side effects.

- **Serving Size:** You can use around 20–40 drops of Asian ginseng up to 3 times per day or drink 1–2 cups of decoction per day. Use 1–2 teaspoons of the ground root with 8 ounces of water to make 1 cup of decoction.

Goji

Lycium barbarum

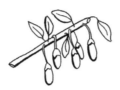

Goji berries grow on a perennial vine and are native to China. They have naturalized in Hawaii, and there is a related species that grows in the southwestern part of the United States. Goji plants aren't especially picky about growing conditions, and do well in average soil with good drainage and full sun. They can be grown in USDA zones 5–9.

In traditional Chinese medicine, liver tonics like goji are often also used to promote the health of the eyes. Goji has a reputation for assisting with poor night vision; dry, red, or painful eyes; glaucoma; macular degeneration; excessive tearing; and cataracts, especially in formulas with other herbs.

This adaptogen is considered a nutritive tonic for the liver, kidneys, and blood, and the antioxidants in goji can help stabilize and strengthen veins, capillaries, and arteries.

- **USDA Plant Hardiness Zone(s):** 5–9

- **Properties:** anti-inflammatory, antioxidant, liver protectant, immune tonic, hypoglycemic, nutritive herb

- **Safety:** Goji is in the nightshade family, so avoid if you have allergies to those plants. Based on traditional use, it may be best to avoid goji if you tend to have diarrhea, flatulence, or bloating.

- **Serving Size:** For goji berry extracts, 60–90 drops of extract can be taken 3–4 times a day. Use 1–2 teaspoons of the dried fruit with 8 ounces of water to make a cup of decoction, or eat up to 1 ounce of the dried fruit per day.

Gotu Kola

Centella asiatica

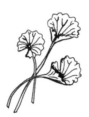

Classified by some herbalists as an adaptogen, and by others strictly as a nootropic (an herb that supports the healthy functioning of the mind), gotu kola is an Ayurvedic tonic herb that is useful for cardiovascular health and as an immune system balancer, thyroid stimulant, and nervous system tonic.

Gotu kola is a wonderful herb to use if you are looking for an adaptogen that supports mental clarity and focus; there have been studies done linking gotu kola with improved neural health for patients with Alzheimer's disease.

One of the most fascinating aspects of gotu kola as an adaptogen is the way that this herb's immune-balancing effects combine with its vulnerary properties. A vulnerary herb is a plant that promotes the health of skin and other tissues throughout the body. Because of this combination of effects, plus anti-inflammatory properties, it appears that gotu kola can be supportive for people struggling with autoimmune conditions such as rheumatoid arthritis, inflammatory conditions of the digestive tract, and allergy-related skin conditions.

Sensitive to frost, gotu kola can be grown in USDA zones 7 and warmer. It needs moist soil and a sunny location. Occasionally I hear from people who are very excited that they found gotu kola growing in their yards, but be aware that there are several look-alikes that can easily be confused with this herb.

According to the current USDA range maps it is only naturalized in Oregon and Florida, so if you think you have stumbled across gotu kola in your yard or garden, check with someone at a local county extension office or seek out an experienced botanist to help you confirm your find.

- **USDA Plant Hardiness Zone(s):** 7–11

- **Properties:** cardiovascular tonic, nervine, thyroid stimulant, immune tonic

- **Safety:** Gotu kola is generally regarded as a nutritive herb with a high margin of safety, even for children. However, gotu kola is rich in constituents known as saponins. Saponins have a number of different actions, but fats and cholesterol are very important for their uptake and utilization in the human body. Because of its saponin content, gotu kola may not be a good choice for people who have fat malabsorption issues, deficiencies in fat-soluble vitamins, or problems with bile production.

- **Serving Size:** A serving of gotu kola is usually around 40–60 drops, and can be repeated up to 3 times a day. To make a tea, 1–2 teaspoons of dried herb can be used in 8 ounces of water up to 3 times per day.

Hawthorn

Crataegus monogyna; Crataegus oxyacantha

Most commonly recognized for cardiovascular benefits, hawthorn also has nervine properties and was used in TCM as a spleen tonic. Herbalist Donald Yance considers it to be an adaptogen, but this is another herb that may or may not qualify as a true adaptogen. Research is beginning to indicate that hawthorn has a wider influence on the body than the cardiovascular system, which is what many people think of when this herb comes to mind.

Although traditionally thought of in the West as a cardiovascular herb, searching a little further back to traditional Chinese medicine brings up many more uses for this herb. As a nervous system herb, hawthorn was utilized for depression, anxiety, and trouble focusing. It also has a record of use as a digestive tonic, in cases where there was bloating, indigestion, or digestive weakness.

Hawthorn is a small tree or shrub that is native to many temperate areas. It can be difficult to identify a hawthorn by the shape of its leaves because they can vary from tree to tree, but hawthorns have characteristic thorns and bright red fruit in the fall. The leaves, flowers, and fruit are all used.

- **USDA Plant Hardiness Zone(s):** 3–9

- **Properties:** digestive aid, cardiovascular tonic, nervine relaxant

- **Safety:** Hawthorn is a very safe herb, and can be used by children as well as adults. It may react with some heart medications to make them more potent, so if you take pharmaceuticals be sure to check with your doctor before using hawthorn.

- **Serving Size:** Serving size for hawthorn is usually 40–60 drops of extract, or 1–2 teaspoons of dried leaves and flowers in 8 ounces of water for a tea, up to 3 times per day.

He Shou Wu (Fo-Ti)

Polygonum multiflorum

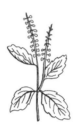

He shou wu means "black-haired Mr. He." Mr. He is credited with the discovery of this herb's properties. There is a lot of fantastic and bizarre lore around this herb if you look back in the ancient literature. (As an example, the root of a 300-year-old he shou wu plant is said to bestow immortality.)

Regardless of some of the wilder claims surrounding this herb in traditional medicine, it is also used for tamer purposes, such as nourishing the kidneys and liver and improving weakness and fatigue, lower back pain, dizziness, insomnia, and erectile dysfunction. It was also used in "hit medicine" formulas that martial artists applied topically. In traditional Japanese herbalism it is used for constipation and inflammatory conditions of the intestines.

Modern applications of the herb are similar; it is used in aiding against dizziness, ringing in the ears, anemia, low back pain, and premature greying. It is also used as a men's fertility herb, and in some cases for women's reproductive health as well.

He shou wu is a flowering vine that is hardy to USDA zone 7. It can tolerate light shade, and prefers sandy, moist soil. It's a perennial, and once established in your garden should come back year after year.

- **USDA Plant Hardiness Zone(s):** 7–11

- **Properties:** antioxidant, astringent, cholagogue (bile flow stimulant), laxative, neuroprotectant, cholesterol reducer

- **Safety:** The unprocessed root of he shou wu can cause diarrhea in some sensitive people. Most he shou wu comes in a prepared form from steaming with black bean juice and yellow rice wine, which makes it less laxative than other forms. It may be best to find an alternative to he shou wu if you have pre-existing liver conditions. Avoid combining this herb with hepatotoxic medications like acetaminophen, tetracycline, and statins.

- **Serving Size:** 30–40 drops of extract 3 times a day. To make a decoction of he shou wu, use 1–2 teaspoons of the dried, cured root per 10 ounces of water. You can drink 4 ounces at a time up to 3 times a day.

Holy Basil (Tulsi)

Ocimum sanctum

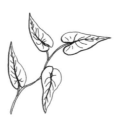

Just as there are different varieties of mint that can be grown in the home garden, there are different types of tulsi. A member of the mint family of plants, there are several types of tulsi that you may encounter for sale as supplements or as garden plants. These include Rama, Krishna, Vana, and Kapoor. These varieties can be used interchangeably, but they have slightly different flavors and aromas. Native to India, parts of China, and many of the surrounding countries, holy basil can be grown as a perennial in tropical areas or as an annual in cooler climates. It can adapt to life as a container plant, and be brought indoors to overwinter.

Tulsi is an Ayurvedic tonic herb that has seen around 3,000 years of traditional use, and is considered one of India's most powerful herbs. In addition to the rejuvenating properties of an adaptogen, folk medicine in India uses the tea as an expectorant for bronchitis and to ease upset stomach and vomiting, and uses the snuff for congestion.

Modern herbalists employ tulsi for the nervous system where there is mental fog, to support memory, to support recovery from head trauma, and as a nervine during depression. Tulsi's immune system properties make it helpful for environmental allergies.

- **USDA Plant Hardiness Zone(s):** 10–11 (may be grown as a houseplant or an annual in other zones)

- **Properties:** nervine, immune system tonic, antioxidant, antiviral, carminative (gas reliever), diuretic, expectorant

- **Safety:** Mixed results in animal studies might mean it is best to avoid holy basil during pregnancy. This herb is traditionally reported to have an antifertility effect, so you should probably avoid this adaptogen if you are trying to get pregnant.

- **Serving Size:** A typical serving size of holy basil is 40–60 drops of extract 3 times a day, or 1 teaspoon of dried herb per 8 ounces of water to make a tea.

Jiaogulan

Gynostemma pentaphyllum

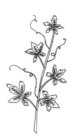

Although there are a few references in older literature about jiaogulan, interest in this herb started in the 1960s, when it was discovered to have several constituents that are identical to those found in Asian ginseng. Even though it has some of the same properties as Asian ginseng, jiaogulan tends to have a calming influence on the nervous system rather than a stimulating one. This member of the cucumber family is weedy and easy to grow, although it is only hardy to around 20°F. It can even be grown in a hanging basket in colder climates and moved indoors for the winter or grown as a houseplant.

Jiaogulan is sometimes also called gynostemma. This adaptogen is excellent as an immune system tonic, and is very high in antioxidants. It can help support healthy cholesterol profiles and improve heart health.

- **USDA Plant Hardiness Zone(s):** 8–11 as a perennial (may be grown indoors or as a container plant in other zones)

- **Properties:** antioxidant, immune system tonic, nervine, liver protectant, expectorant

- **Safety:** Be careful when combining jiaogulan with blood thinners, tranquilizers, or sedatives, as there is a potential for this herb to interact with these medications. Try taking this herb with food to minimize the chances of an upset stomach. If you take too much of this herb, you might experience palpitations, fatigue, dizziness, or a rash.

- **Serving Size:** A serving of jiaogulan extract is usually 80–120 drops, up to 3 times a day. To make a tea, 1–2 teaspoons of the herb may be used in 8 ounces of water and taken up to 3 times a day.

Licorice

Glycyrrhiza glabra

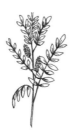

As an adaptogen, licorice has antiviral, antihistamine, anti-inflammatory, antioxidant, and expectorant properties. It is an excellent immune tonic, and can help balance the immune system when it is over- or underactive. It's also a good herb for digestive tract health, assisting when there are conditions present with too much inflammation.

This herb is also traditionally used as a liver-protective herb to help the liver process and handle exposures to toxins, or to offer support from drug- or virus-induced liver damage. Licorice is often used in small amounts in classical Chinese herbal formulas, as it was believed to act as a harmonizer of all of the herbs in the formula.

Native to southeastern Europe and southwestern Asia, licorice prefers warm climates such as USDA zones 7–10, and appreciates a sunny spot with well-drained soil. It can grow to a height of 5 feet, so make sure to provide it with a spot where it has enough room.

- **USDA Plant Hardiness Zone(s):** 7–10

- **Properties:** immune system normalizer, anti-inflammatory, liver protectant

- **Safety:** Many traditional Chinese herbal formulas include a small amount of licorice, and it might be best to consider the same or a similar approach when using licorice in the present day. Large amounts of licorice over an extended time can cause the body to retain sodium, lose potassium, and develop high blood pressure—a condition known as hyperaldosteremia. If you have high blood pressure, licorice may not be a good choice. Licorice also doesn't combine well with diuretics that deplete potassium, certain kinds of antidepressants, or digoxin.

- **Serving Size:** A serving of licorice extract may be as low as 10 drops up to 3 times a day, or range up to 60 drops 3 times a day. If you intend to use licorice long term, stay to the lower end of the range and discontinue use if you notice signs that your electrolytes are getting off balance (such as water retention or muscle cramps) or high blood pressure.

Maca

Lepidium meyenii

Maca is a root vegetable grown in Peru, and is unusual in that it manages to thrive under the incredibly harsh growing conditions of the high elevations in the Andes Mountains. Although there is much interest in maca as a functional food and it is widely believed to be an adaptogen, tracking down human studies to confirm the potential actions of maca can be difficult. For the most part, it is valued for increasing libido and hormonal health in men and women, although the exact way that it does this is not understood. Some research has been done into the different varieties of maca (there are eight different types), and this work does show that each type has a slightly different profile of vitamins, minerals, and other factors. Although it is used as a vegetable in Peru, it is only available in a dried and powdered form in the United States. Maca may be grown in some areas of North America, although it may be difficult to do so in most places. Maca needs a cold climate and high altitude.

- **USDA Plant Hardiness Zone(s):** N/A

- **Properties:** aphrodisiac, nutritive tonic, sperm count booster

- **Safety:** Maca is traditionally used as a food so it is widely regarded as safe, but there is little research to date that has yielded information on potential drug interactions.

- **Serving Size:** Generally, maca supplements will suggest a serving size starting at 1,000–1,500mg of maca powder per day, usually divided into several servings.

Nettle

Urtica dioica

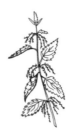

Nettle is most widely known for its nutritious leaves that make a lovely foraged green and that support lung and kidney health as well as immune system health during allergy season. Less well known are the benefits of nettle root, which is used to support prostate health, and nettle seeds, which are used in traditional Chinese medicine to support health of both the prostate and the kidneys. Herbalists Kiva Rose and Henriette Kress both write about their experiences with nettle seed as an adaptogen. According to Rose, nettle seed can promote increased energy, reduce stress, and assist with mental clarity. According to Kress, nettle seeds are a potent kidney tonic and trophorestorative. In herbalism, trophorestoratives are nourishing herbs that have a particular affinity for supporting a specific organ system. Another example of a trophorestorative is hawthorn with its affinity for the heart. Nettle seeds help support the body's response to stress and strengthen the function of the adrenal glands just as well as other more exotic adaptogens.

Like burdock, which is discussed earlier, there's nothing at all exotic about this adaptogen, which is one of the things I find the most wonderful about it. It's weedy, wild, and can be grown in most climates. The leaves do pack a nasty sting thanks to tiny, hollow hairs that contain formic acid, so you will need to wear gloves when harvesting nettles. The sting soon leaves nettles once they have dried or wilted. Young leaves are also boiled to get rid of the sting before being eaten. Despite the temporary sting, nettles are considered very safe to use when prepared correctly.

If you want to utilize nettle seeds, chances are you will need to grow your own, because most sources that offer the seeds only offer the amount that comes in a seed packet for gardening.

- **USDA Plant Hardiness Zone(s):** 2–10

- **Properties:** kidney and adrenal tonic

- **Safety:** While wearing gloves, rub the seeds through a sieve to get rid of the sting and allow them to dry.

- **Serving Size:** Kress suggests using 1–2 tablespoons of the seed in yogurt or thick juice. They can also be added to soups and stews or used as a seasoning on food. Kiva Rose prefers making an extract with the fresh seeds, and notes that as little as 1–5 drops may be effective, or that a full serving of 30 drops may be used. A serving of nettle seeds can be used up to 3 times a day.

Reishi

Ganoderma lucidum

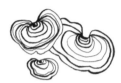

Reishi is a very mild adaptogen that needs to be taken over a longer period of time in order for it to express its full benefit. A great deal of research on reishi has been done over the years. This herb seems to be beneficial for the cardiovascular system, has nervine properties, and supports liver health.

As an immune system tonic, reishi acts as an immunomodulator, a substance that can either increase or decrease immune system activity depending on what is needed for the immune system to achieve balance. It is also being studied for potential use as immune system support during cancer treatment.

There are actually six types of reishi listed in traditional Chinese herbalism, and each variety is believed to have slightly different qualities. Reishi mushrooms can be grown indoors using medicinal mushroom grow kits available from specialty suppliers.

- **USDA Plant Hardiness Zone(s):** N/A

- **Properties:** antiviral, heart tonic, immune system tonic, nervine

- **Safety:** Reishi is usually considered a very safe adaptogen, and one that can be used long term.

- **Serving Size:** 80–100 drops of extract can be taken up to 6 times a day.

Rhodiola

Rhodiola rosea

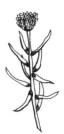

This adaptogen is a succulent that grows in cool, northern climates. It is native to Canada, Russia, and Scandinavian countries. It grows best in full sun and dry, sandy soil or a rock garden.

Rhodiola is part of the official Russian pharmacopoeia as an antidepressant and nerve tonic. Traditionally, this herb was used to increase mental stamina and physical endurance, to boost the immune system during winter, and as a fertility and endocrine tonic for men and women.

Like eleuthero, rhodiola can help support the immune system in athletes, as hard training can sometimes cause a decline in immune function. Rhodiola may also help balance blood sugar levels, help with fertility and reproductive health in both sexes, strengthen the heart, and protect the heart from stress-related damage. Another name for rhodiola is roseroot.

- **USDA Plant Hardiness Zone(s):** N/A

- **Properties:** antiviral, nervine, immune stimulant, heart tonic, neuroprotectant

- **Safety:** Rhodiola can cause insomnia if taken too late in the day, and it may be best to avoid using rhodiola if you have mental health disorders.

- **Serving Size:** A serving of rhodiola extract is generally in the range of 40–60 drops, and can be taken 3 times per day. For a tea, 1–2 teaspoons of the dried root can be decocted in 8 ounces of water and used up to 3 times per day.

Schisandra

Schisandra chinensis

Schisandra berries, the part of the plant used in herbalism, are known as the "five flavor" fruit, and the taste definitely lives up to that unusual moniker. If you hold a dried berry in your mouth for a few minutes, you will quickly realize that different parts of the fruit are responsible for the different flavors. The peel is sweet, sour, and a little salty, but when you bite into the seeds you will unleash the bitter and pungent tastes.

Although schisandra is generally considered a calming adaptogen, it actually has a double effect on the nervous system. Besides being calming and helping to relieve anxiety, it also enhances reflexes and concentration.

A traditional use for schisandra is to help dry up excessive fluids, so it was sometimes used for diarrhea, frequent urination, wet coughs, and reproductive problems like premature ejaculation or copious vaginal secretions.

- **USDA Plant Hardiness Zone(s):** 4–7

- **Properties:** antioxidant, astringent, expectorant, immune tonic, nervine

- **Safety:** According to traditional usage, schisandra should not be taken during acute illnesses.

- **Serving Size:** For extracts, 40–80 drops at a time up to 4 times a day may be used. To make a tea, 1–2 teaspoons of the berries are decocted in 8 ounces of water, and 4 ounces of the tea may be taken up to 3 times a day.

Shatavari

Asparagus racemosus

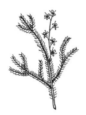

Mentioned in the Rig-Veda, which dates back to 1500 B.C.E., shatavari is a type of wild asparagus used extensively in Ayurveda. The name of this herb has two possible translations, thanks to homonyms in the original Sanskrit: "She who has hundreds of husbands" or "One hundred roots." Both names are surprisingly fitting. Shatavari is a beloved herb for women's health and fertility, and has a mass of thick, succulent roots below the deceptively thin stems above ground. Besides being used as an aphrodisiac and women's tonic, shatavari is also useful as a tonic when there is fatigue and poor appetite. It is traditionally used for inflammation of the bladder and urethra as well as irritable coughs with sticky mucus. Its soothing, demulcent properties make it useful for urinary, respiratory, and digestive health.

In its native range, shatavari can be found in India, Southeast Asia, Malaysia, Africa, and even northern Australia, and is suited to USDA zones 8–11. Shatavari appreciates full sun but can grow in part shade, and has a climbing growth habit suited to its native forest habitat. The roots are the portion of the plant used in herbalism, but the tender young sprouts can be cooked and eaten as a vegetable.

- **USDA Plant Hardiness Zone(s):** 8–11

- **Properties:** antispasmodic, diuretic, immune tonic, lung tonic, lactation stimulant

- **Safety:** Generally considered to be a very safe herb with few, if any, side effects or drug interactions, shatavari does have mild diuretic properties that could intensify the effects of pharmaceutical diuretics or interfere with prescription medications that are excreted through the kidneys.

- **Serving Size:** Shatavari extract can be taken up to 3 times a day, in a serving size between 40–80 drops at a time. For a tea, 2 teaspoons of the herb are usually decocted in 8 ounces of water and taken up to 2 times per day.

Suma

Pfaffia paniculata

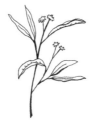

Suma is a rainforest herb with the Spanish nickname *para todo*, which means "for all things." It's also sometimes called Brazilian ginseng, although it is not part of the Araliaceae family at all. It's actually related to amaranth and quinoa. Like maca, suma has received a lot of attention in the past several years as a potential adaptogen, but was mostly used as a traditional food.

- **USDA Plant Hardiness Zone(s):** N/A

- **Properties:** Currently, suma is a potential adaptogen whose ethnobotanical and pharmacological activities have yet to be fully explored. Speculative benefits of suma include boosting sexual performance and libido, enhancing immune function, supporting the endocrine system, and increasing energy levels. Bodybuilders sometimes use suma with the belief that compounds in this herb (beta-ecdysterone) mimic testosterone and will help increase muscle mass.

- **Safety:** Potential safety issues pertaining to suma are currently unknown.

- **Serving Size:** A serving size of suma appears to be in line with most other adaptogenic herbs, with powdered herbs and tablets starting at 1,500mg, 2 times a day, and liquid supplements usually starting at a range of 30–40 drops up to 4 times a day.

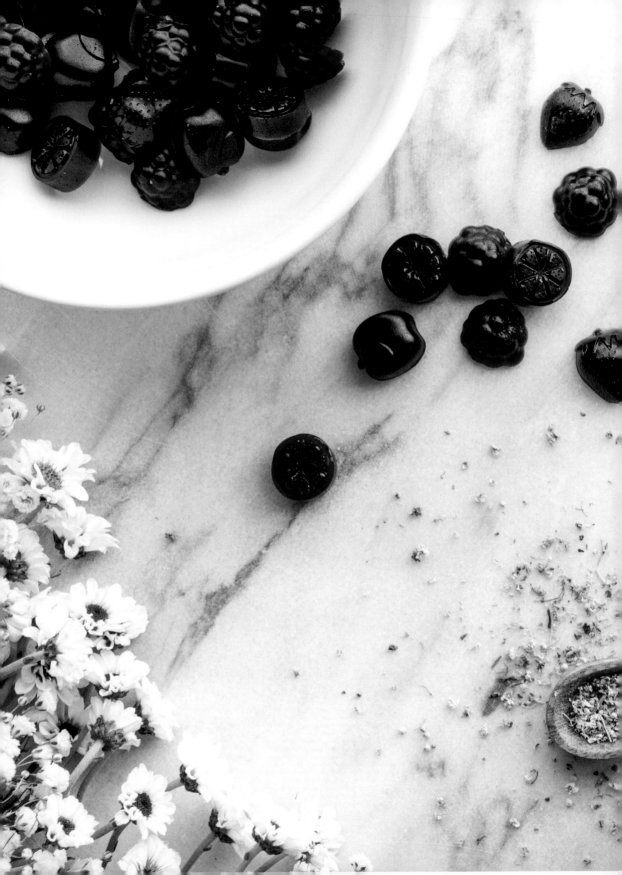

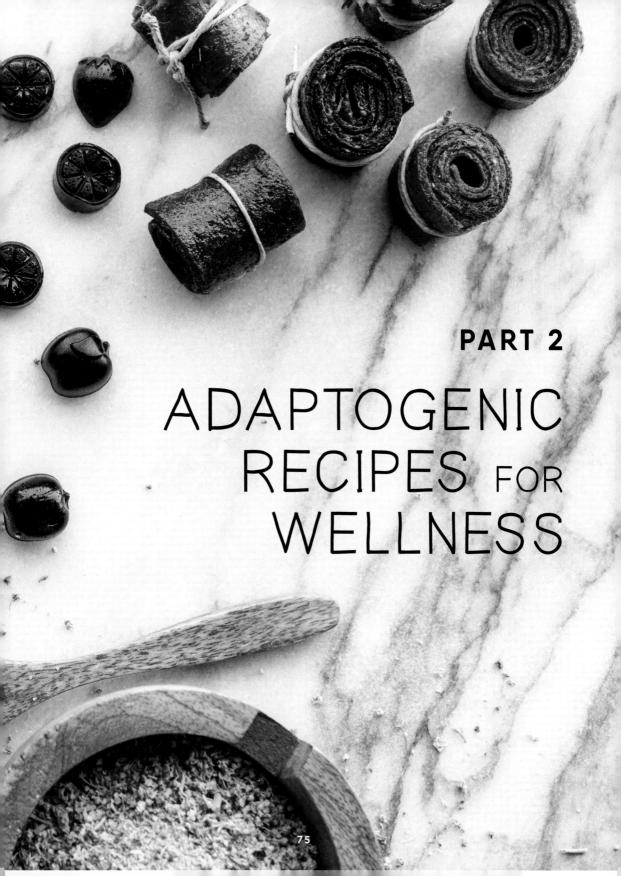

PART 2
ADAPTOGENIC RECIPES FOR WELLNESS

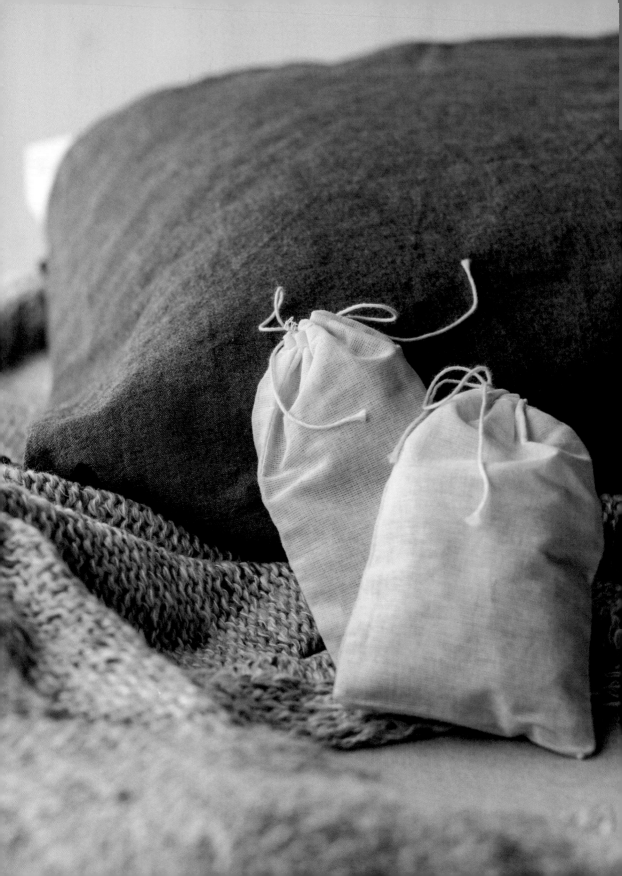

CHAPTER THREE

RECIPES TO IMPROVE YOUR SLEEP

Without proper sleep, the rest of your health quickly suffers. Some adaptogens are too stimulating to be part of a bedtime routine, but others may be perfect to help support a good night's sleep. Pay attention to how your body responds to each recipe or adaptogen you try, because no two people will respond exactly the same way to any herb. You may find that certain adaptogens work best for you, or that you need to adjust the timing of when you take them (either closer to or further from bedtime to give them a chance to work). The recipes in this section are meant to help support a healthy bedtime routine, but you need to make sure you aren't fighting them. It may be helpful to create a calming bedtime routine, turn off screens and electronics an hour before bed, and make sure your bedroom is a place you associate with comfort and rest.

Another class of herbs, called nervines, complement the actions of adaptogens and can safely be used alongside them. Nervines help support the health of the nervous system in many ways. Chamomile is a well-known nervine that is often used to help soothe away stress after a long day, but other nervines, like lemon balm and linden, can be used either before bed or during the day. Nervines that are especially helpful as part of a bedtime routine because they are known to promote a good night's rest include hops, valerian, and California poppy.

Simply Schisandra and Rhodiola Extract

Like eleuthero, rhodiola can help support healthy sleep, but rhodiola tends to have a more energizing influence during the day. Add schisandra's supportive nervine abilities to the mix, and the result is an unusual and useful combination to help you power through the day but still give you an easier time winding down at night. It's definitely best to take this extract during the earlier part of the day, so make sure your last serving of this extract is before 4:00 p.m.

Rhodiola can help your body adapt to interruptions in your circadian rhythms, and gives a nice boost to overall sleep quality. Although it's great as a sleep support blend at home, because rhodiola can help your body adapt to the stress of altitude changes it may be an extract to remember when you are traveling too!

How to Make

Combine both extracts in a 4-ounce amber glass bottle. Label the bottle with the ingredients and the date. A serving of this extract is 30–60 drops.

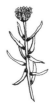

YIELDS 4 OUNCES (ENOUGH FOR 1 MONTH)

2 ounces rhodiola root extract
2 ounces schisandra berry extract

Midnight Milk

It's best to avoid using most adaptogens late in the day because they can give the body a boost of energy right when it should be getting ready for sleep. Ashwagandha, on the other hand, is a very calming, soothing adaptogen that can be taken right up until bedtime.

Milk and dairy products such as clarified butter are often used in Ayurvedic herbalism because milk is said to help bring out the nutritive aspects of herbs used with it. If you wish to avoid cow's milk, you can try this recipe with goat's milk or a plant-based milk such as coconut or almond.

Not known for having a pleasant taste, ashwagandha is paired here with more flavorful rose, a nervine that complements the calming actions of ashwagandha, and spices to round out the flavors. Schisandra berry is another adaptogen, and one that has been used traditionally for dream-disturbed sleep.

The first step to make Midnight Milk is to blend together a batch of Midnight Milk Powder.

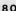

Midnight Milk Powder

YIELDS 60 SERVINGS

¼ cup powdered ashwagandha
¼ cup powdered schisandra berries
1 cup powdered rose petals
1 teaspoon ground cinnamon
1 teaspoon ground nutmeg

How to Make

Blend together all the ingredients and store in an airtight container in the pantry until you are ready to use.

Midnight Milk

YIELDS 1 SERVING

1 cup milk or plant milk
¼–1 teaspoon Midnight Milk Powder
Honey, to taste

How to Make

1   In a small saucepan, heat 1 cup of milk until warm. Be careful not to scald or cook the milk.

2   Pour the milk into a mug, and stir in ¼–1 teaspoon of Midnight Milk Powder (as desired).

3   Sweeten with a little honey, and drink in the evening or as part of a bedtime snack.

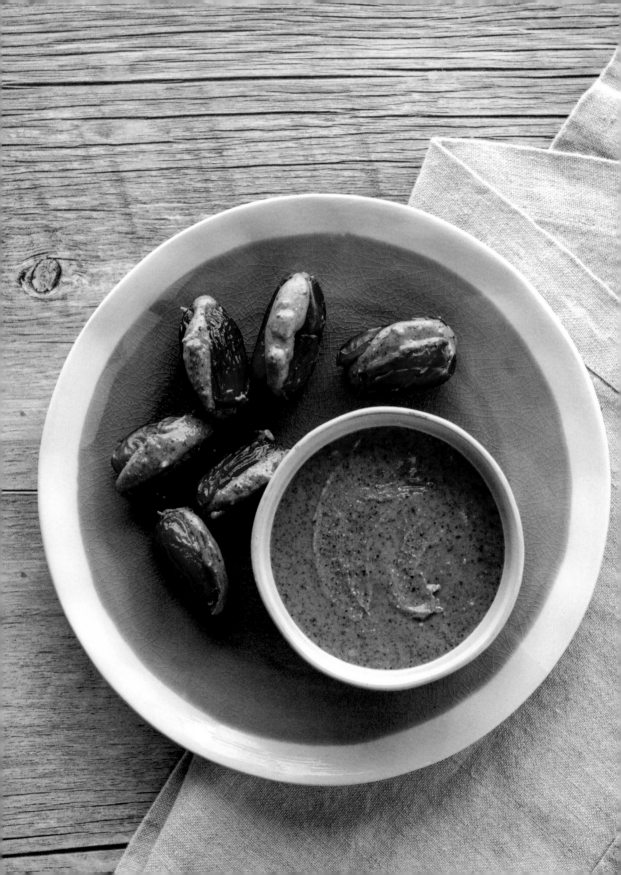

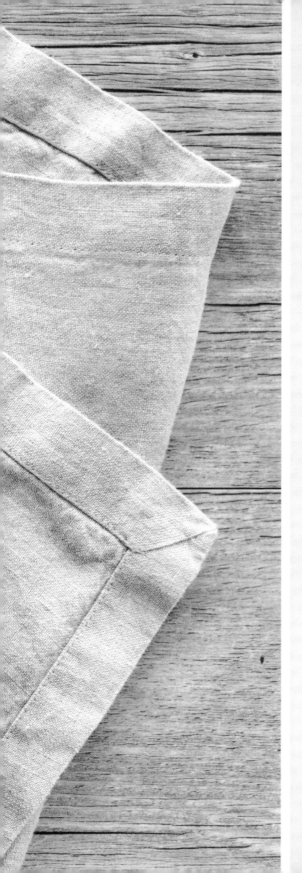

Bedtime Nut Butter Bites

These quick and simple bedtime snacks are a sweet treat rich in calcium and magnesium, and support a good night's sleep even without adaptogens. Add almond butter mixed with Bedtime Spice for an extra boost of sleepytime goodness.

In traditional Chinese medicine, schisandra berry is considered to be more soothing and grounding, and less stimulating, than many other adaptogens. Unlike its more energizing counterparts, schisandra's effect is said to be one of calming the heart and quieting the spirit.

In this recipe, an adaptogen blend featuring schisandra is mixed into nut butter and used as a stuffing for dates, but it can also be eaten with crackers, apple slices, or a bagel half—anywhere you would normally enjoy a bit of nut or seed butter.

The first step to make Bedtime Nut Butter Bites is to blend together a batch of Bedtime Spice.

Bedtime Spice

YIELDS 48 SERVINGS

7 tablespoons powdered schisandra berries
5 tablespoons powdered ashwagandha
3 tablespoons powdered chamomile

How to Make

Blend together the powdered schisandra berries, ashwagandha, and chamomile in a small mixing bowl. Transfer to an airtight container and store in the pantry until you are ready to make Bedtime Nut Butter.

Bedtime Nut Butter

YIELDS 1 SERVING

1 teaspoon Bedtime Spice
1 tablespoon almond butter (or other nut butter)

How to Make

1 Combine 1 teaspoon Bedtime Spice with 1 tablespoon almond butter in a small bowl.

2 If you would like to make a larger batch, use 5 tablespoons Bedtime Spice per cup of nut or seed butter and blend well, until the herbs are evenly mixed in the spread.

3 Store Bedtime Nut Butter in the refrigerator until you are ready to use it.

Bedtime Nut Butter Bites

YIELDS 3 STUFFED DATES

3 pitted dates
1 tablespoon Bedtime Nut Butter

How to Make

1   Slice open each date to make a pocket for the Bedtime
    Nut Butter mixture.

2   Stuff each date with $\frac{1}{3}$ tablespoon of Bedtime Nut Butter
    mixture. Enjoy!

How Do You Know an Herb Is Still Good?

If you've had a dried herb sitting in your pantry for a few
months, how do you know it's still good? You should famil-
iarize yourself with the way your herbs look and smell when
they first arrive. Using a reputable supplier helps boost the
chances that your herbs will be fresh and vital when they
arrive. Herbs will have unique smells and a unique appearance. Anything that starts to look dull and nondescript and
has lost its smell is probably well on its way out. Sometimes
a batch might get buggy or moldy, so keep an eye out for
that. Mold can sometimes be seen visually—a dried herb
may seem dustier than normal when you give the container
a shake—or sometimes it will be detectable in a smell. The
best way I know to describe a moldy herb smell is that it is a
little musty and has a distinct peppery aroma.

Morpheus Tea Blend

Jiaogulan takes center stage in this tea blend, as much for its flavor and natural sweetness as for its calming, nerve-nourishing abilities. Why the funny name for this blend? In ancient Greek mythology, Morpheus is the god of dreams and the son of the god of slumber. Two nervines, hops strobiles and linden flowers, round out the traditional actions of gynostemma, and are also popular bedtime herbs. Although chamomile is a time-honored nighttime tea, I find that sometimes it gives me uncomfortably vivid dreams. If you notice a similar pattern, lemon balm may be a good choice instead. Dried lemon balm won't alter the flavor profile very much in this recipe, but fresh lemon balm will. Jiaogulan's natural sweetness pairs well with dried apple pieces and cinnamon in this tea.

When you are using this blend to make a tea, feel free to sweeten the tea if you desire. But test it first; you may find that the tea is sweet enough on its own, as jiaogulan and chamomile both have a natural sweetness, and of course the apple pieces do as well.

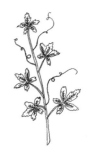

**YIELDS APPROX.
20 SERVINGS**

2 tablespoons powdered
   jiaogulan
1 tablespoon powdered
   chamomile
1 tablespoon linden
   leaves and flowers
½ tablespoon hops
   strobiles
1 cinnamon stick
2 tablespoons diced
   dried apple pieces

How to Make

1 Combine jiaogulan, chamomile, linden leaves and flowers, and hops in a large glass mixing bowl.

2 Gently pound the stick of cinnamon with a mortar and pestle to break into small pieces; add the cinnamon pieces to the mixing bowl of herbs.

3 Add the apple pieces to the mixing bowl with the herbs and cinnamon, and stir with clean hands or a wooden spoon to blend all ingredients together.

4 Transfer to an airtight container, and store in a cool, dark pantry away from light and humidity.

A Cup of Morpheus Tea

YIELDS 1 (8-OUNCE) CUP

1–2 teaspoons Morpheus Tea Blend
8 ounces hot water

How to Make

1 Place 1–2 teaspoons of Morpheus Tea Blend into a tea strainer, filter, or bag.

2 Fill your favorite mug or teacup with 8 ounces of hot water just off the boil, and add the strainer or filter with the Morpheus Tea Blend.

3 Cover with a saucer and allow to steep 10 minutes before removing the saucer and strainer.

4 Allow to cool to a comfortable warm temperature before drinking. Sweeten if desired.

Harvesting Leaves and Flowers

Linden is a perfect example of an adaptogen that is grown for its leaves. But how do you know when it's ready to harvest? Most of the time, the leaves should be harvested at the peak of growth right before a plant blooms. After they bloom and set seeds, most herbs are spent for the year. The aerial portions of the plant will usually start to die back. In annual plants, this marks the end of the plant's life. In biennial plants and perennials, the focus of the plant's energy becomes building up the root system for fall and winter. If you test a leaf by rubbing it between your fingers every few days throughout the growing season, you will also notice the plant's smell becoming stronger as it gets closer to bloom. By harvesting just before the flowers blossom, you will capture all of those volatile oils and compounds at their peak.

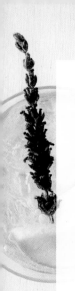

Powdering Cut and Sifted Herbs

So what happens if a recipe calls for a powdered ingredient, but all you can find in stock through your regular resources is cut and sifted? Cut and sifted means that the herb has been cut into roughly same-sized pieces and anything smaller gets sifted out. With leaves, that means the final product is little leaf flakes. With roots, that means the final product looks like a fine gravel. These are definitely a far cry from powdered. As long as you have a coffee grinder, though, you can make your own powdered herbs from cut and sifted. Just remember to work with only a tablespoon or two of herbs at a time and not let your coffee grinder overheat. I've only had to give up on one batch of roots that I was powdering in this way. It was some asclepias root (butterfly weed) that I was using for a respiratory formula. They were too hard and dense for the coffee grinder and it started to overheat. A coffee grinder can handle most herbs and roots just fine!

Sandman's Reserve Elixir

This elixir is a good travel blend, or nice to have on hand when you want to enjoy the benefits of adaptogens without spending much time in the kitchen. The good thing about elixirs as a whole is that they are more palatable than regular extracts. With Sandman's Reserve Elixir, you can take ¼ teaspoon as is, or stir it into a small glass of water to sip as you get ready for bed.

Part of the fun of working with elixirs is the artistry that goes into developing a pleasant taste for the finished product. Sometimes this is done by adding spices and flavorings like vanilla or cinnamon, but you can also experiment with different types of brandy and honey to create a blend that you find particularly pleasing.

Like extracts, elixirs don't need to be refrigerated, so you can keep a bottle of Sandman's Reserve Elixir on your nightstand or in your travel bag to have close by when you need it!

How to Make

1   Combine the ashwagandha, rose petal, skullcap, chamomile, and linden powders in a clean, dry glass canning jar. You can stir them or blend them together if you like, but you will be shaking the jar once you add the brandy, so it isn't necessary.

2   Pour the brandy on top of the herbs, and place the lid on the jar.

3   Shake gently to combine, and allow to infuse for at least 2 weeks in a cool, dark cupboard.

4   Check the jar with the herbs and brandy daily to make sure that the herbs stay submerged in the alcohol. Add more brandy if needed to keep the herbs submerged.

5   At the end of 2 weeks, filter the herbs from the brandy and measure the extract to determine how much you have. It should be around 4 ounces, but this can vary based on how much alcohol the herbs absorbed and how much alcohol was left in the herbs when you strained them. Add an equal amount of honey, and stir gently until the honey and extract are combined.

6   Transfer the elixir to a clean, amber glass bottle with cap, and make sure to label and date your creation. Most elixirs will be shelf stable at room temperature for at least a year, thanks to the preservative powers of the honey and the brandy.

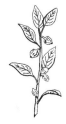

YIELDS 8 OUNCES
(48 SERVINGS)

2 tablespoons
   powdered
   ashwagandha
1 tablespoon powdered
   rose petals
1 tablespoon powdered
   skullcap
½ tablespoon
   powdered chamomile
½ tablespoon
   powdered linden
   leaves and flowers
5 ounces brandy
4–5 ounces honey

Night Garden Sachets

These herbal sachets rely on a class of herbs that are complementary to the actions of adaptogens: nervines. Traditionally used to heal and support the health of the immune system, nervines include some of nature's most wonderfully aromatic plants. Owing in part to their volatile oil content, these aromatic nervines have a reputation for soothing and calming even through scent. Lavender and rose combine for a floral blend, but by using thyme instead of rose the impression becomes fresh and woodsy, reminiscent of a night outdoors.

The scent of these herbs comes from the presence of volatile oils, one of the same compounds that make essential oils effective for aromatherapy. As the herbs are crushed from the weight of your head and warmed by your body heat, a little more of the fragrance is released each night. Even though you might think that something as insubstantial as a smell could not possibly have an effect on your body, the scent molecules are actually connecting and binding with receptors in your body and being absorbed into your bloodstream through your lungs. Aroma can be a subtle but effective healing tool.

Over time, the fragrance will fade away and you will need to refresh the herbs in your sachets. If you notice a musty smell, that's also a good indication that the herbs need to be replaced with a fresh batch. Trust your nose!

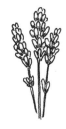

**YIELDS 1 CUP
OF DRIED BLEND
(16 TABLESPOONS)**

8 tablespoons dried
rose petals or thyme
leaves
4 tablespoons dried
hops
4 tablespoons dried
lavender buds
2 (4" × 6") muslin
drawstring bags

How to Make

1 Combine all herbal ingredients in a medium mixing bowl.

2 Fill one drawstring bag with herbs and tie the bag shut. Place the filled, tied bag upside down inside the other bag to prevent any herbs from spilling out as the sachet is used, and tie the second bag closed.

3 If there is leftover herb blend in your mixing bowl, transfer it to a labeled airtight container in the pantry so you can refresh your sachet when it begins to lose its scent.

4 Tuck your sachet into the pillowcase of your bed pillow. Whenever you notice that the scent of your sachet has faded, you should refill it with fresh herbs.

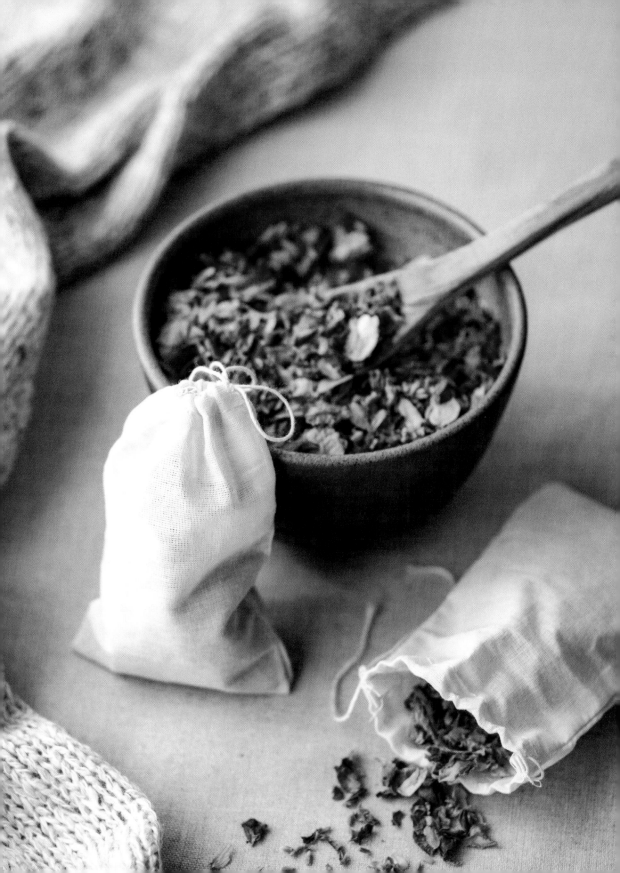

Soothed Spirits Bath Blend

An evening bath is a before-bed ritual that calms, warms, and soothes. Holy basil is a calming adaptogen with nervine properties, but in Ayurveda, it is also believed to have an effect on the chakras, the subtle energy centers of the body. By combining it with sage and mugwort, two Western herbs with similar cleansing reputations, this evening bath becomes a ritual of calming the body and mind while cleansing and balancing the spirit. Please note that this blend may not be appropriate during pregnancy.

If you don't have a tub for taking a bath, you can use 4 tablespoons of this blend to create a foot soak for a relaxing alternative. Mugwort was traditionally used as a traveler's herb to soothe tired feet and legs, so this can also be a nice way to unwind after a long day on your feet. To make a foot bath, use the second method in step 4 for brewing a bath tea, and then add the bath tea to your foot basin. A foot basin can be any bowl or basin large enough for your feet and enough water to reach your ankles. Since you will be using it for herbal foot soaks, try to find a nonreactive glass or ceramic bowl rather than one made of metal.

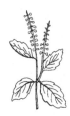

YIELDS ENOUGH FOR 6 BATHS

1 cup cut and sifted holy basil leaves

1 cup cut and sifted garden sage (*Salvia officinalis*) leaves

1 cup cut and sifted mugwort leaves

Large glass canning jar or decorative, airtight container

1 quart water

How to Make

1   Place holy basil, sage, and mugwort in a large mixing bowl and stir gently with a wooden spoon or clean hands to combine.

2   Transfer to a large glass canning jar or decorative, airtight container that suits your bathroom decor.

3   When you are ready to take a bath, you have two ways to proceed. In the first method, you would transfer ¼ cup of Soothed Spirits Bath Blend to a clean muslin pouch and hang it from your tap by the drawstrings. Position the bag so that the hot water for your bath flows over the bag. When your bath has been drawn, remove the pouch and allow it to steep in the water with you while you bathe.

4   In the second method, you would brew a quart of strong infusion in a nonreactive saucepan. Bring 1 quart of water to a boil, and add ¼ cup Soothed Spirits Bath Blend. Replace the lid on the pot and allow to steep for 20–30 minutes. Filter out the herbs, and add the infusion to your bath just before you step in. A bath made using this second method is typically stronger than one made with the first method; you may find you have a personal preference for one or the other.

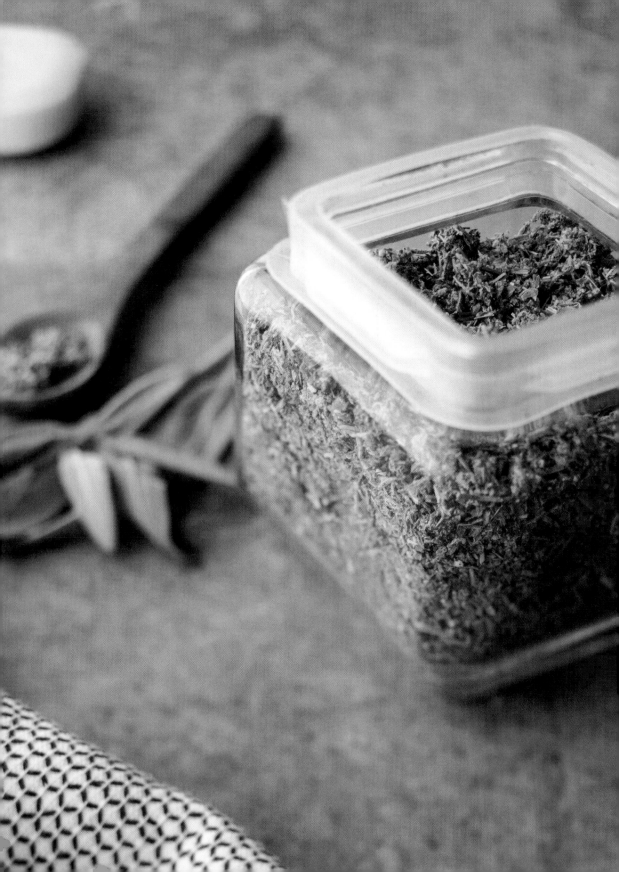

Night Nectar

This recipe for Night Nectar combines two adaptogen powders, ashwagandha and schisandra, with honey to create a blend worthy of sweetening your evening tea, spreading with nut or seed butter on your nightly nibble, or drizzling over apple pieces for a bedtime snack.

Ashwagandha is a calming adaptogen that works well when used at night. It can help soothe sleeplessness when one of the main factors behind it is high stress levels. Schisandra has nervine properties that calm and focus the nervous system. An interesting and less well known aspect of schisandra is that it can be used when there is insomnia or waking caused by vivid or unpleasant dreams.

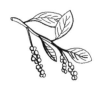

YIELDS 16 SERVINGS

3 tablespoons powdered schisandra
3 tablespoons powdered ashwagandha
1 cup honey

How to Make

1   Place schisandra and ashwagandha powders in a clean mixing bowl and stir gently until they are evenly combined.

2   Measure 1 cup of honey into a glass canning jar. Place the jar in a small saucepan with enough water to come a quarter of the way up the outside of the jar.

3   Warm the honey over low heat until it flows easily off of a spoon, and immediately remove the jar from the water using an oven mitt or canning jar lifter. (Too much heat will cause the honey to crystallize, and all you want to do by warming it is to make stirring in the herbs easier.)

4   Before the honey cools, add the schisandra and ashwagandha mixture and fold gently to combine evenly as the honey returns to room temperature.

Harvesting Roots

If you've decided to grow adaptogens like dang shen (codonopsis), rhodiola, or ashwagandha in your own garden, you may be wondering about when to harvest roots. Typically, roots are harvested in the fall. The age of the plant can matter too. Some herbs may be fine to harvest for their roots after the first or second year of growth, but others may need many years before the root system has grown enough for harvest. Ashwagandha can be grown as an annual in much the same way as tomatoes in many areas (they are actually related!), so you plant the seeds in the spring and then harvest the plants in the fall for the roots. Other herbs, like ginseng, need at least five or six years before they reach full maturity and strength.

Night Nectar and Fried Banana Bedtime Snack

"Moth broth" is something you might remember from school science fair projects when you were a kid. Essentially, if you make a paste with bananas and other ripe fruit, sweeten it with sugar, and paint it on a tree at dusk you have a fascinating way to observe some of the velvety denizens of the night.

While it won't attract any moths for you to observe, this fried banana treat made with the Night Nectar adaptogen might just become one of your favorite adult bedtime snacks. Although you might not have an annual entry in the science fair anymore, nobody really outgrows a bedtime snack.

YIELDS 1 SERVING

1 medium under-ripe
  banana
1-2 teaspoons coconut
  oil
1 tablespoon Night
  Nectar
1 tablespoon water

How to Make

1   Prep the banana by peeling it and slicing into coins.

2   Heat coconut oil in a small skillet over low heat and arrange the banana slices in the skillet so they can cook.

3   Allow to cook about 2 minutes on each side, or until they are golden.

4   Whisk the Night Nectar and water together in a small cup.

5   Take the skillet off the heat and pour the Night Nectar and water mixture over the bananas. Enjoy while still warm.

Better Rest Elixir

Sometimes better sleep can be had when you support your nervous system during the day, rather than waiting until the last minute before bedtime. Studies with eleuthero have shown that taking it through the day can help promote healthy sleep at night. Eleuthero is usually considered a calming adaptogen, but if you are very sensitive and find that eleuthero gives you a bump in energy, you might prefer to take your last serving of this extract before 4:00 p.m. Take it 2 or 3 times a day, whichever frequency works best for you.

The addition of eleuthero in this blend makes it particularly useful when you are trying to reset your sleeping rhythms after traveling and may be struggling with jet lag. Eleuthero is believed to help you sleep through the night without waking and to make your overall quality of sleep improve.

How to Make

1   Combine the eleuthero powder and ashwagandha powder in a medium bowl. If you are making a percolation extract, moisten the herbs with a little extra vodka and prepare the glass funnel according to the directions in the project "Make an Herbal Extract by Percolation" in Chapter 1.

2   After allowing the vodka and herbs to rest overnight, adjust the screw cap on the funnel until you achieve one drop every 1–3 seconds. Let the extract percolate, then discard the remaining herbs.

3   Measure the finished extract, and combine it with an equal amount of honey by volume. Bottle in an amber glass bottle with a label describing the ingredients and the date. A serving is ¼–½ teaspoon up to 3 times a day.

YIELDS APPROX.
4 OUNCES
EXTRACT
(48-96 SERVINGS,
ENOUGH FOR
1 MONTH)

½ ounce eleuthero
    powder (by weight)
½ ounce powdered
    ashwagandha (by
    weight)
5 ounces vodka

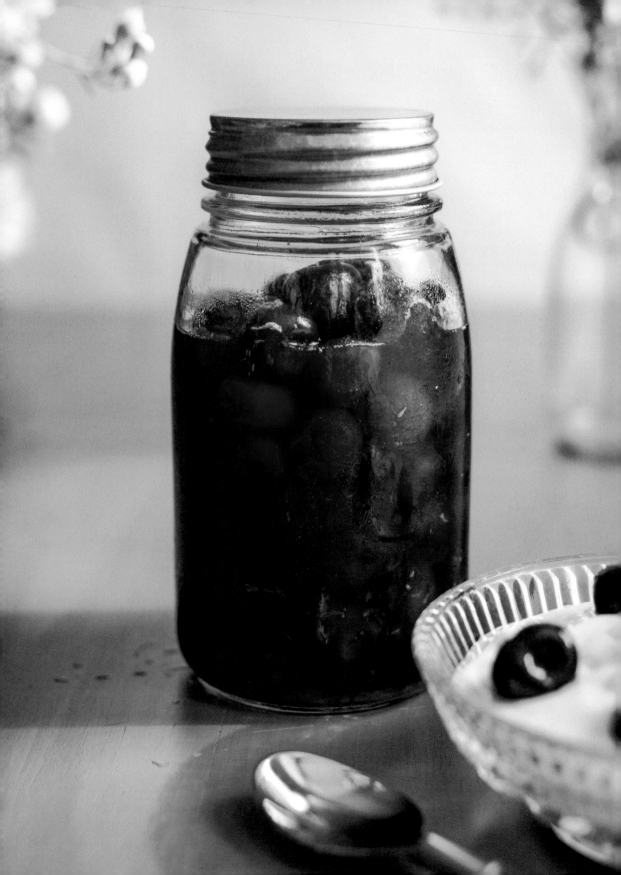

Thyme for Sleep Berries and Cherries

These brandied cherries include the adaptogen schisandra. Thyme adds an unusual note to the brandied cherries, while having calming nervine properties of its own. Use a few cherries and schisandra berries at a time over desserts or added to yogurt for a bedtime snack. When the berries and cherries are all gone, use ½ teaspoon of the remaining liquid as an unusual evening elixir.

Even though it's usually thought of simply as a kitchen spice, thyme has an impressive number of herbal attributes. It offers support to the digestive system as a carminative (an herb that helps to soothe gas and bloating), and to the lungs as an antitussive and expectorant.

Thyme's history as a nervine is virtually unknown, but I find it particularly fascinating because of its affinity for the nervous system. At various points in history it has been employed for everything from anxiety to epilepsy to paralysis to fainting. In sleep support formulas, it can be a good choice to promote relaxation from subconscious sources of tension and restlessness in someone who can be easily startled awake or who has nightmares.

How to Make

1   Pack the cherries and schisandra berries into a quart-sized canning jar or divide evenly into smaller jars.

2   Heat the brandy, sugar, and thyme in a medium saucepan over low heat until the sugar dissolves.

3   Pour the brandy and sugar mixture into the jars to cover the cherries. Place lids on the jars, and transfer to the fridge for at least 1 week. The berries and cherries should keep indefinitely as long as they are kept covered by the brandy and sugar solution and refrigerated.

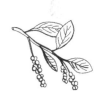

YIELDS 1 POUND BRANDIED BERRIES AND CHERRIES

15 ounces frozen cherries (fresh are also nice, but remember to remove the pits and stems)

1 ounce dried schisandra berries

2 cups brandy

½ cup granulated cane sugar

1 teaspoon dried thyme

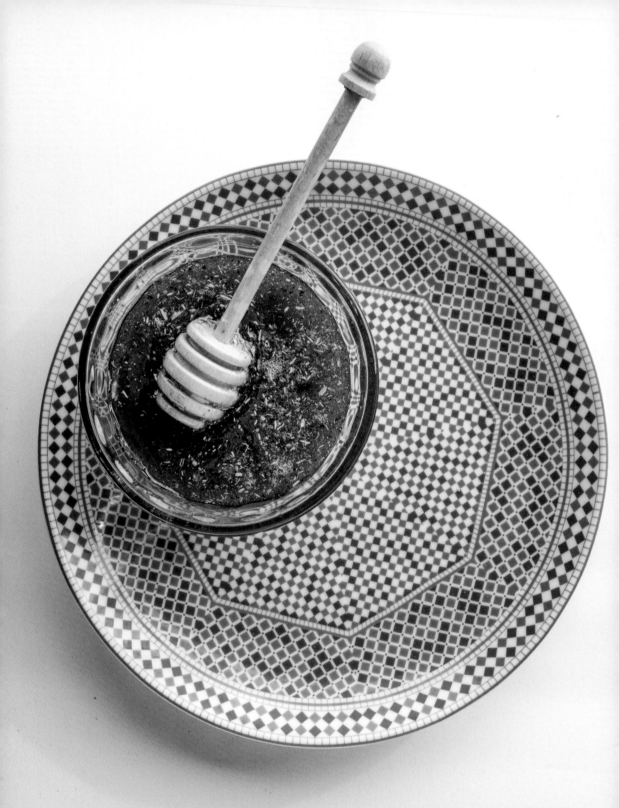

CHAPTER FOUR

RECIPES TO IMPROVE YOUR MOOD

Many different factors can influence our mood and over-all sense of well-being. Simple things like getting enough quality sleep, eating a well-rounded selection of nutritious foods, and getting enough physical activity can make a big difference in our emotional outlook. Herbs can help move us in the right direction by supporting the health of our central nervous system and our emotional well-being.

There are several different classes of herbs that can help support emotional well-being. We've already mentioned nervines in several recipes throughout the book. Not only do some adaptogens also have nervine properties, but they generally pair very well with other nervine herbs.

"Nervine" is a broad category of herbs and it helps to break them down by their secondary actions to understand them a little better. Some are hypnotic (they help promote sleep), some are relaxants that help ease tension in the body, and some are tonics that help balance the nervous system.

In addition to nervines and adaptogens, there's another category of herbs known as nootropics that can help with mood and the health of the mind. "Nootropic," translated from its Greek roots, means "acting on the mind." These herbs help support the brain and mental processes more directly than a nervine. Lavender, which is used in some of the recipes in this chapter, is an example of an herb that is both a nervine and a nootropic.

Happy Days Elixir

Three adaptogens combine in a blend that is actually equally at home being used as an uplifting mood tonic, an athlete's elixir, or support for the immune system. A serving of Happy Days Elixir is 40–80 drops, up to 3 times a day. If this elixir interferes with your sleep schedule, use it in the mornings only.

Rhodiola and eleuthero are excellent for the dragging energy levels that can go along with a not-so-happy mood. Rhodiola has the added benefit of having an uplifting influence on the mood. Because it focuses the nervous system and calms anxiety, the schisandra in this blend can be good for those days when you feel scattered and out of sorts, and maybe a little worked up emotionally.

How to Make

1   Combine the powdered rhodiola, eleuthero, and schisandra in a glass jar, and pour in the brandy.

2   Screw on the lid of the jar, and gently shake to combine all of the ingredients.

3   Allow the brandy and herbs to blend for 2 weeks. Shake the jar every day, and add more brandy if the herbs absorb it all. There should be enough brandy in the jar to keep the herbs covered at all times so that they don't dry out.

4   After 2 weeks, strain out the powdered herbs and add in the honey. Bottle and label your elixir. Store in a cool, dark place.

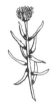

YIELDS 8–10 OUNCES

⅓ ounce powdered rhodiola root
⅓ ounce eleuthero powder
⅓ ounce powdered schisandra berries
5 ounces brandy (by volume)
5 ounces honey (by volume)

Tulsi Agua Fresca

Tulsi is a sacred herb in India, and traditional as well as modern herbalists value it for an uplifting action on the mood and balancing influence on the nervous system.

This recipe calls for fresh tulsi leaves. There are three main types of tulsi plants or seeds available through special order nurseries. Kapoor is the most common, and Vana and Rama are the other varieties. Each one has a different flavor profile, but they can be used interchangeably (both in this recipe and in others).

Making a Tulsi Agua Fresca works best if you have access to the fresh plant. If you don't have fresh tulsi leaves available, you can make a tea with dried leaves—chill it in the refrigerator with the fruit and enjoy a refreshing tulsi iced tea instead.

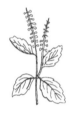

YIELDS 2 SERVINGS

1 quart filtered or
distilled water (for
best taste)
½–1 cup diced seasonal
fruit of your choice
2–4 teaspoons fresh tulsi
leaves, sliced thin

How to Make

1   Fill a quart-sized pitcher with filtered or distilled water.

2   Place the ½–1 cup of chopped fruit into the pitcher of water.

3   Gently bruise the sliced tulsi and add it to the pitcher of water.

4   Give your agua fresca a stir and let it steep in the fridge for at least 4 hours or overnight.

5   Pour into a tall glass and sip it throughout the day as a naturally flavored water. Discard any leftovers after 2 days.

Sparkling Herbal Refreshers

Herbal fizzes and refreshers are a fun way to enjoy adaptogens. These work best when they have a taste that you enjoy, so feel free to experiment with different adaptogens and flavoring herbs. The recipes here focus on combining adaptogens and nervines to make a pleasant drink to enjoy during times when you are feeling stressed or want a fun and uplifting beverage.

To make an herbal fizz, you need seltzer. Seltzer is plain water with added carbonation—no other ingredients. You can experiment with club soda (which has added minerals) or sparkling mineral water (which generally comes from a natural spring or well), but both of these will add a different dimension of flavor to the finished drink. You will generally want to stay away from tonic water for these recipes, as it contains quinine, sweeteners, and other ingredients. Really, though, the type of sparkling water you decide to use is up to you. For the simplest taste profile, go with plain seltzer.

You will also need herbal extracts, because although you can use a tea with a sparkling water, you end up diluting both the seltzer and the tea, resulting in what may or may not be a particularly satisfying experience. For each glass of sparkling water, you should use a single serving of extract, which is usually defined as 30–60 drops. Be sure to follow the suggested serving size on any herbal supplements you purchase from the store.

Be careful not to use essential oils in your fizz. You need the alcohol-based extracts, sometimes also called tinctures. Essential oils are an entirely different preparation, and they are far too concentrated to use in this recipe. Essential oils should not be mixed in drinking water—the oils are not water soluble and form a film that sits on the top of the water and can cause damage to the sensitive tissues that line your mouth, throat, and stomach.

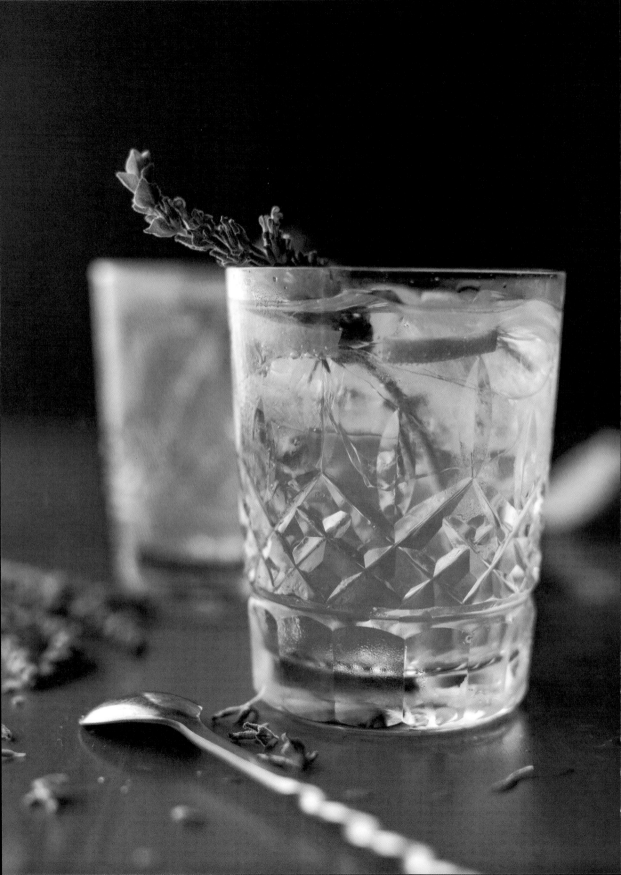

Lavender Tulsi Sparkling Water

The only ingredients needed to make this refreshingly simple seltzer are lemon, lavender, and tulsi. Tulsi excels at offering emotional support during particularly stressful days or when you are feeling a little down.

The flavors of lavender and lemon complement each other beautifully. When combined with lemon, which always seems to be an uplifting taste to me, I think lavender does a very nice job clearing and acting as an emotional "reset" button. It helps that lavender is also a nervine and nootropic for emotional well-being.

How to Make

1   Pour the sparkling water into a glass. This will be the base of your drink.

2   Add the serving of tulsi extract and the 5 drops of lavender extract. Stir with a spoon to disperse the extracts into the water.

3   Squeeze the lemon wedge gently over the glass and drop it into your drink. Garnish with a sprig of fresh lavender buds, if desired.

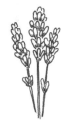

YIELDS 1 (12-OUNCE) SERVING

12 ounces sparkling
    water
1 serving tulsi extract
    (usually around 30–
    60 drops, depending
    on the brand)
5 drops lavender extract
    (not essential oil or
    lavender flavoring)
1 lemon wedge
1 sprig fresh lavender
    buds (optional)

Albizia Fizz

This unusual seltzer calls for albizia extract, rhodiola extract, and rose water. Albizia has a reputation among herbalists as a mood tonic that is especially suited to grief or deep sadness. If you can, use an albizia extract made with only the flowers. It will have a milder, more floral taste than one that also contains the bark. The flowers and bark are commonly combined to make an extract, so go with what you are able to find. If you have an albizia tree growing in your yard, you may find it worth your while to make your own extract with only the flowers.

Strawberries, raspberries, or blackberries all go well with this drink, as do peaches or plums—simply add a finely chopped strawberry, a few lightly crushed raspberries or blackberries, or a slice or two of a plum or peach to the glass to add extra flavor.

YIELDS 1 (12-OUNCE)
SERVING

12 ounces sparkling
    water
15–30 drops albizia
    extract
15–30 drops rhodiola
    root extract
1 tablespoon rose water
Fresh fruit (optional)

How to Make

1 Pour the sparkling water into a drinking glass. This will be the base of your drink.

2 Stir in the albizia extract, rhodiola root extract, and rose water.

3 If desired, drop in the fresh fruit of your choice for extra flavor: fresh strawberries, raspberries, blackberries, peaches, or plums. Enjoy!

Vine and Berry Tea

Jiaogulan and schisandra berries make an elegant cup of tea. Jiaogulan tastes a bit like a sweeter version of nettles, and schisandra berries have a complex flavor that's difficult to describe. Combining berries and leaves in a tea requires a little more work than simply using leaves, because berries need a bit longer to steep.

How to Make

1 Bring 10 ounces of water to a boil in a medium saucepan and add the schisandra berries.

2 Simmer the berries for 10 minutes, then remove from the heat and allow them to steep for 20 minutes. The decoction will have reduced a little while it simmered, so you should now have around 8 ounces remaining.

3 Bring the berries and tea back to a simmer and add the jiaogulan leaves. Remove the tea from the heat, and allow it to steep for 10 minutes. Strain the tea and sweeten it as desired.

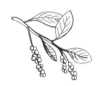

YIELDS 1 (8-OUNCE) SERVING

10 ounces water
1 teaspoon dried
    schisandra berries
1 teaspoon dried
    jiaogulan leaf

To Caffeinate or Not?

What do you want to hear—that coffee and other caffeinated beverages are amazing and good for you, or that they are bad for you? Well, chances are you can find someone with a convincing argument either way. I love my caffeine, too, but let's face it: it's a stimulant. You can't get around that fact. Too much can leave you sleepless, wired, and anxious. With enough of it, you could also upset your stomach and elevate your heart rate. Dependency can be an issue with regular use, and withdrawal can cause headaches and irritability. On the positive side, caffeine can help you stay alert when you need to, may boost memory and improve mood, and is full of antioxidants. So basically we should probably approach it with mindfulness and not overdo it. All things in moderation except moderation!

Rhodiola and Rooibos Latte

Who doesn't enjoy a nice latte as a pick-me-up or a treat now and then? Skip the caffeine, and get a boost from rhodiola and rooibos instead!

Rhodiola can help reduce cortisol levels (one of the hormones our body produces when we are under stress), and can give a boost to "feel good" brain chemicals like dopamine, so it's perfect for a good-mood latte.

Rooibos has a lovely taste that I think goes very well with rhodiola, and has many health benefits of its own. Sometimes called red tea even though it's not related to the plant that gives us black and green tea, rooibos comes from South Africa and is rich in minerals and antioxidants.

Together they give you a nutritious latte with a little extra love for your emotional well-being.

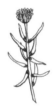

YIELDS 1 (12-OUNCE) SERVING

2 teaspoons dried
  rhodiola root
6 ounces water
8 ounces plant milk
  (rice, nut, or soy)
2 rooibos tea bags
Sweetener of your
  choice: honey, maple
  syrup, or sugar

How to Make

1 Roots need a little longer to brew to make a good tea, so begin by placing the rhodiola into a small saucepan with the 6 ounces of water. Bring to a boil and allow to simmer with the lid on for 20 minutes.

2 Once the rhodiola has brewed for 20 minutes, it's time to add the other ingredients. Turn off the heat. Stir in the plant milk of your choice, and add the rooibos tea bags.

3 Allow the rooibos tea bags to steep for an additional 5 minutes, then strain the latte through a mesh strainer into your favorite mug.

4 Add your sweetener to taste and enjoy!

Rooibos

Looking for an energizing but caffeine-free herbal
tea? Rooibos is worth a try. Rooibos comes from
South Africa and is rich in vitamins and minerals
with a pleasant, complex taste. Rooibos comes in
either red or green varieties, just like *Camellia
sinensis*—the herb most people are thinking of when
they say, "tea."

Uplifting Massage Oil

For Uplifting Massage Oil, you will need to learn the technique for infusing dried herbal material into an oil. Unlike adding a few drops of essential oil to a carrier oil, creating an infused oil takes a little more time but is well worth the effort. This blend utilizes both techniques: infusing the carrier oil with rhodiola, and then adding a few drops of frankincense essential oil. Frankincense is one of my favorite essential oils for emotional well-being. If you have a personal favorite, you might wish to substitute it instead.

For this recipe, I use 3–6 drops of essential oil per ounce of carrier oil. This is what the National Association for Holistic Aromatherapy suggests as a safe 0.5–1 percent solution for sensitive skin (my skin is very sensitive). This dilution rate also makes sense because the rhodiola root is the main star of this blend, and the essential oil plays a supporting role.

I favor sesame or olive oil for this blend over other common carrier oils such as grapeseed or almond oil, because I find they hold up better with the low heat processing that's necessary to make an herbal infused oil.

You can use either powdered rhodiola root or cut and sifted root. I like using the powdered root because the oil is better able to coat and extract from the smaller particles of herb (there's more surface area available!). If you go with powdered herbs, a cloth strainer on a stand like the ones used for jelly making make straining a simple procedure. Otherwise you will end up with flecks of powder in your massage oil, which is a little uncomfortable!

Following are two options for making your infused oil. If you would like the oil to be done in a day, you can use a double boiler to heat the oil at a consistent temperature for 4 hours. The drawback is that you need to stay close by to monitor the oil, since the stove will be on. If you don't mind waiting for a few weeks, you can let the oil infuse at room temperature. Without the heat, it will need to infuse around 4–6 weeks for best results, but you won't need to babysit it during that time. To use your oil, pour a teaspoon at a time into the palm of your hand and allow it to warm up with your body heat. Use it for a self-massage on your feet, arms, legs, or neck and shoulders.

YIELDS 1½-2 CUPS

½ cup powdered rhodiola root
2 cups olive oil or sesame oil
3-6 drops essential oil per ounce of carrier oil (24-48 drops total)

How to Make the Done-in-a-Day Version

1 Combine ½ cup powdered rhodiola root and the olive or sesame oil in a double boiler. If you don't have a double boiler, pour the herb and oil into a large canning jar, and place the jar into a medium saucepan. Pour water into the saucepan (not into the jar with the oil and herbs) until the saucepan is about half full. Turn on the burner to medium heat so that the saucepan or double boiler provides a steady, consistent temperature for the infusing oil.

2 Use a thermometer to check the temperature of the oil periodically. You want it to stay in the range of 100–140°F. A thermometer with a temperature alert setting can be helpful.

3 Allow the oil to infuse for around 4 hours in the target temperature range, then remove the oil from the heat and allow it to cool completely.

4 Use a muslin cloth in a colander over a bowl or a jelly-making bag on a stand to strain the herbs out of the oil.

5 Measure your essential oil drop by drop into the bowl of infused oil. Stir gently to combine.

6 Pour your oil into an airtight bottle or jar and label clearly, "For external use only." Make sure to store your oil out of direct sunlight.

How to Make the Longer Version

1 Although there is a longer wait time for this version of the oil, it doesn't require supervision once the oil and herb have been mixed.

2 Combine the rhodiola and olive or sesame oil in a glass canning jar. Screw on the cap to keep the oil clean.

3 Place the jar into a brown paper bag to block direct sunlight, and find a spot in a sunny window to keep the oil for the next 4–6 weeks. Sunlight can degrade the oil and the herbs, but the warmth of the sun will help the herbs infuse into the oil.

4 At the end of 4 weeks, or 6 weeks if you can be that patient, strain the herbs out of the oil. Add your drops of essential oil to the infused oil. Stir gently to combine. Then bottle the oil. Label clearly, "For external use only."

Mexican Chocolate Goji Berries

Although they seem like a decadent treat, chocolate-covered goji berries couldn't be easier to make, and adding cayenne and cinnamon gives this easy treat a distinctive flair. If you don't care for Mexican-style chocolate, feel free to leave one or both of the spices out.

Dark chocolate can be a nice, mood-boosting treat. It's been shown to raise levels of endorphins and serotonin (brain chemicals that are important for staying in a good mood). Goji has traditionally been used to support mood and well-being. Both chocolate and goji are full of antioxidants too!

I like these as an alternative to chocolate-covered raisins, and they make a great trail mix ingredient.

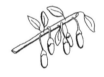

YIELDS 4 SERVINGS

1 cup dark chocolate
  baking chips
¼ teaspoon cayenne
  pepper
¼ teaspoon ground
  cinnamon
1 cup dried goji berries

How to Make

1 Melt the chocolate baking chips in a small saucepan over low heat, stirring gently, until the chocolate is smooth.

2 Sprinkle in the cayenne and cinnamon and stir gently to combine.

3 Add the goji berries and stir until they are evenly coated with the chocolate.

4 Use a slotted spoon to transfer the chocolate-covered goji berries to a baking sheet lined with waxed paper.

5 Once the chocolate has cooled and hardened, transfer the chocolate-covered goji berries to an airtight container. If you plan to enjoy them within a few weeks they can be stored at room temperature; otherwise, you might want to store them in the freezer.

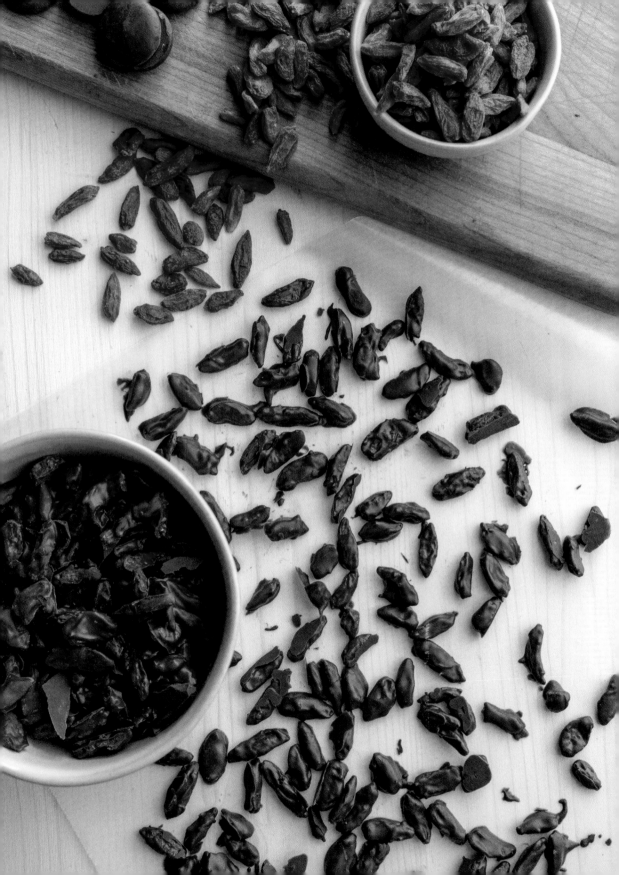

Small Measure of Calm Honey

Small Measure of Calm Honey is an example of an herbal electuary: a simple blend of herbs and honey that can be used as a sweetener in food or tea, or enjoyed a dab at a time just as it is!

Holy basil is included in this recipe because it is an uplifting adaptogen. Schisandra is also uplifting and provides support for the nervous system. Both herbs have a reputation for putting a damper on anxiety and letting happiness have a chance to step to the front for a bit. Goji berries add antioxidants and mood support to the blend.

This honey paste is perfectly suited to herbal snack time. Made with powdered goji berries, schisandra berries, and holy basil, it can be stirred into hot tea, mixed with nut butter and spread onto crackers or bread for a fancy herbal PB and Honey, added to yogurt, or used as a dip for fruit. If you want a vegan option, try rice syrup or agave syrup.

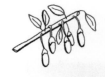

YIELDS 1 CUP
(1 SERVING IS
1-2 TEASPOONS)

2 tablespoons powdered
  goji berries
2 tablespoons powdered
  schisandra berries
2 tablespoons powdered
  holy basil
1 cup honey

How to Make

1 Stir together goji berries, schisandra berries, and holy basil in a small glass mixing bowl to create an evenly blended powder.

2 Once the powdered ingredients have been combined, add 1 cup of honey to the mixing bowl and combine well with the herbal ingredients.

3 Transfer the finished electuary to an airtight container and store in a cool pantry or the refrigerator. It should keep for at least 6 months, but I usually try to use it up by 3 months for the sake of freshness.

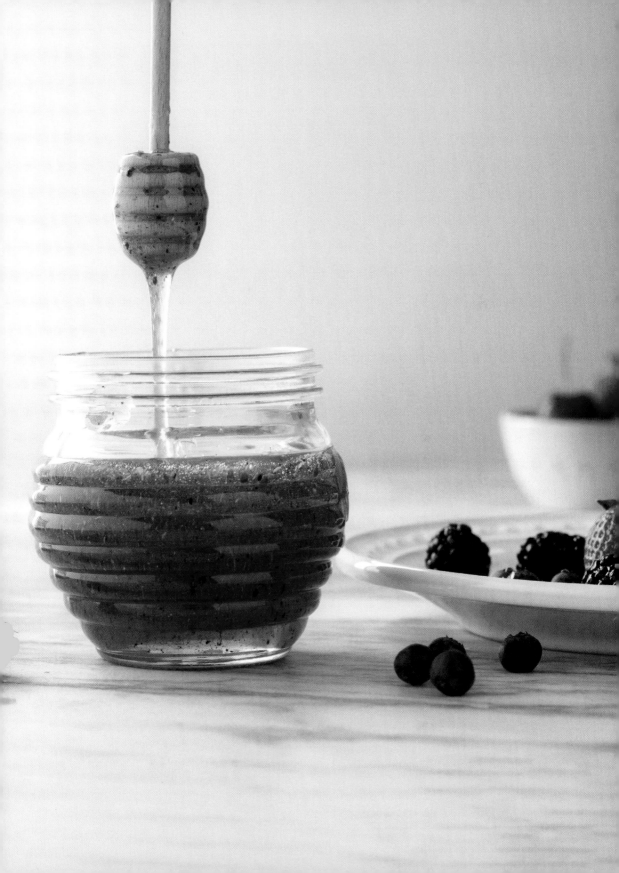

Savor the Day Spice and Fig Morsels

Schisandra is an unusual herbal pick-me-up that can help support emotional well-being. It has a very distinctive flavor that is somewhat resinous and bitter, sour, and sweet all at once. Rosemary, a nervine that has been studied for mood-enhancing properties, adds another unique savory note to these schisandra and fig morsels. When combined with your favorite nut or seed butter, the result is a sophisticated nibble. If the figs don't provide enough sweetness for your liking, I suggest a bit of maple syrup with these.

Interestingly, rosemary has a reputation for benefiting the mind and brain that goes all the way back to the 1600s! Modern studies are beginning to confirm some of these traditional uses, and finding that even just the scent of rosemary may be enough to support better memory. Rosemary is also an uplifting herb that's good for diffusing trapped emotional energy when you feel frustrated and stuck in a mood that you just can't shake.

Savor the Day Spice

YIELDS 24 SERVINGS

1 tablespoon powdered rosemary
6 tablespoons powdered schisandra berries

How to Make

1   Combine the powdered rosemary and powdered schisandra berries and store in an airtight container until ready to use.

2   A serving size is $1/2$–1 teaspoon if used in cooking, or $1/2$ teaspoon if making the Fig Morsels.

Fig Morsels

YIELDS 1 SERVING

¼ teaspoon Savor the Day Spice
1 tablespoon nut butter of your choice
5 dried figs
Drizzle maple syrup (optional)

How to Make

1   In a small bowl, combine ¼ teaspoon Savor the Day Spice and 1 tablespoon of your favorite nut butter.

2   Slice open your figs and divide the nut butter and herb blend evenly between them, making 5 little fig sandwiches.

3   If you like, drizzle each fig bite with a bit of maple syrup.

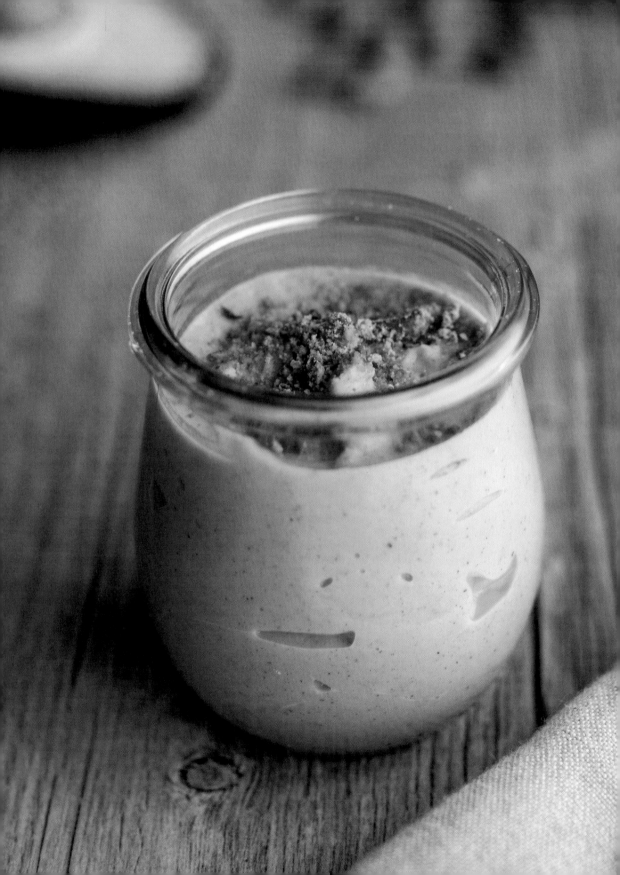

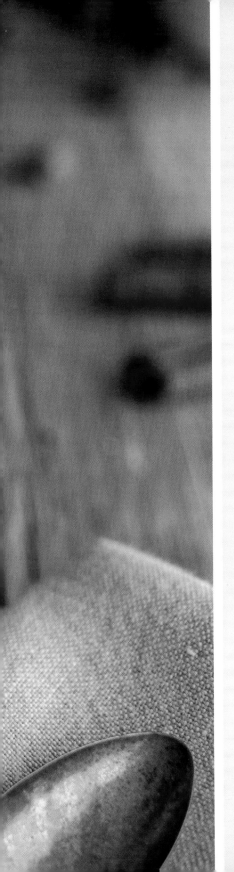

Pistachio Avocado Pudding with Sweeter Mood Spice

Avocados are my favorite snack. Most people never get past guacamole with these little green gems, but if that's you, I have to tell you—you're missing out! Why not try a sweet and simple dessert-style pudding made with avocado instead? Add a dash of Sweeter Mood Spice for some adaptogenic mood support. This recipe makes a single serving of pudding, but you can easily double the recipe if you want to share. Use whatever milk or plant milk you like best. A vanilla-flavored milk is especially nice!

The two adaptogens in this blend, rhodiola and ashwagandha, provide the all-around resiliency that make adaptogens so valuable. Ashwagandha supports emotional well-being with a calming influence, and rhodiola can give a cheery boost to your outlook on life.

The first step to make this dish is to blend together a batch of Sweeter Mood Spice.

Sweeter Mood Spice

YIELDS 24 SERVINGS

3 tablespoons ground cinnamon
2 tablespoons powdered rhodiola root
1 tablespoon powdered ashwagandha
1 tablespoon ground ginger
1 teaspoon ground nutmeg

How to Make

1   Combine all powdered herbs and spices in a bowl, stirring gently until they are evenly combined.

2   Transfer the Sweeter Mood Spice blend to a small airtight container until you are ready to use it. Remember to label your creation so you can easily find it later.

Pistachio Avocado Pudding with Sweeter Mood Spice

YIELDS 1 SERVING

1 medium ripe avocado
1 teaspoon Sweeter Mood Spice
½ cup milk or plant milk
Honey, agave, or maple syrup, to taste
¼ cup crushed pistachio pieces, for garnish

How to Make

1   Spoon the avocado flesh into a blender or food processor along with the Sweeter Mood Spice and the milk. Blend until smooth.

2   Taste the mixture to determine how much sweetener you would like to add.

3   Once the pudding is sweetened to your liking, transfer it to a serving bowl. Sprinkle the pistachios on top, and enjoy!

Mind-Body Connection

Sometimes a bad mood isn't just a bad mood. In herbalism especially, we like to acknowledge that the physical body can influence
the emotional state—and vice versa! In fact, in traditional Chinese
herbalism, there are five emotions in particular that are associated
with specific organs. So an herbalist will sometimes look for patterns in the health of an organ to help balance the corresponding
emotion, or look to the presence of extended or extreme emotional patterns to help understand the potential disharmony within
an organ system. Examples include fear and anxiety, which can
indicate an imbalance with the kidneys; grief, which is associated
with the lungs; anger, which ties in with liver health; chronic worry
or overthinking and the health of the spleen; and overexcitement
and imbalances in heart health. Of course, this is just one aspect
of understanding emotional health, so it's important to seek out
the support and resources that you need. Whether that means
talking with an herbalist, a counselor, a medical professional—or
a combination of all three—you deserve a happy and balanced
emotional life!

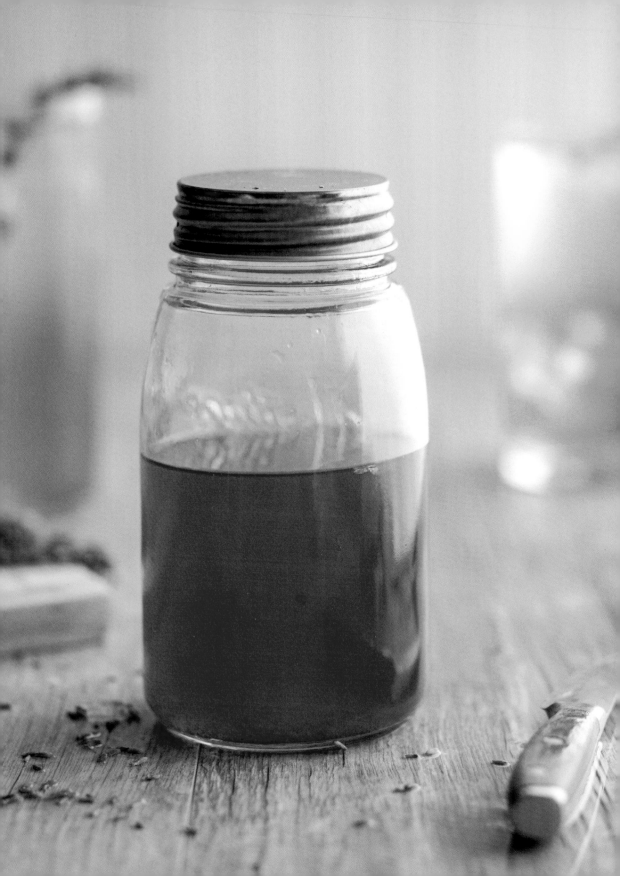

CHAPTER FIVE

RECIPES TO IMPROVE YOUR MENTAL FOCUS

The influence of adaptogens on the mind and mental abilities ranks alongside immunity and physical stamina as one of their most popular potentials. Most of them appear to offer at least some form of support for the mind, although the kind of support varies from one adaptogen to another.

Adaptogens such as ginseng, ashwagandha, dang shen, eleuthero, rhodiola, and schisandra are all believed to support overall brain function and mental clarity. In studies, it seems that some adaptogens have a positive effect on the amount and quality of mental work that subjects complete.

Adaptogens like jiaogulan and cordyceps help support the central nervous system, while other adaptogens can offer more specific support when neurological problems come into play.

Adaptogens can have either a stimulating or a calming effect on the mind and mental processes. Asian ginseng and American ginseng are examples of adaptogens that stimulate the mental processes. Ashwagandha, cordyceps, and jiaogulan are known for being relaxing. Schisandra, on the other hand, is a bit of both. Other adaptogens may not have a noticeable stimulating or calming effect, but still enhance memory and learning.

A class of herbs known as nootropics seem to have a pronounced influence over cerebral function and combine beautifully with adaptogens. Well known nootropics include bacopa, ginkgo, gotu kola, lavender, and rosemary. Although it is typically less familiar to everyday lay herbalists, white peony root (*Paeonia lactiflora* syn. *P. albiflora*) is another nootropic that supports memory, and is included in a few recipes throughout this book.

This chapter includes recipes for snacks, elixirs, and teas that make great accompaniments to work or study. Just remember not to burn the candle at both ends! Make sure you are supporting your brain with enough sleep, good food, and time for fun and relaxation instead of forcing yourself to run full steam ahead without a break in sight. Whip up a few of these snacks to have handy in the fridge or pantry when you need a mental boost.

Cinnamon Candied Walnuts with Eleuthero

So what makes good brain food? Nuts are pretty good mental fuel, thanks to selenium and other trace minerals and protein. Walnuts, in particular, have a high level of DHA, an omega fatty acid. Omega-3s are essential fatty acids that support the permeability of cell membranes in the brain and help your neurons communicate better!

Adding a little eleuthero to the spice blend brings adaptogens to the brain food party. This recipe comes together quickly once the nuts are toasted, so it's an easy one to make even if you only have a few minutes to spare.

This recipe makes 4 servings. These candied walnuts are great on their own, or you can add them to a trail or snack mix, use them to top yogurt or a fruit salad, or even pair them up with crackers and cheese.

YIELDS 4 SERVINGS

1 cup walnut halves
1 tablespoon butter
¼ cup sugar
½ teaspoon ground
   cinnamon
1 teaspoon eleuthero
   powder

How to Make

1   Scatter the walnuts in a single layer on a baking sheet and toast in a 350°F oven for around 10 minutes, or to the level of toastiness that appeals to you. Once the walnuts are toasted to your liking, remove them from the oven and set them aside. This step enhances the flavor of the finished nuts and the texture, but if you prefer your walnuts raw you can skip this step.

2   While the walnuts toast, prepare a second baking sheet by lining it with a piece of parchment paper.

3   Place the butter and sugar into a medium-sized frying pan or saucepan over low heat. Use a spatula or wooden spoon to stir these two ingredients continuously until they have melted.

4   As soon as the ingredients have liquefied, sprinkle in the cinnamon and eleuthero while you continue to stir, so that the spices are evenly distributed in the sugar mixture.

5   Work quickly and stir the toasted walnuts into the mixture. Stir gently and continuously until they are evenly coated.

6   Spread the sugar-and-spice-coated walnuts onto the baking sheet lined with parchment paper.

7   Use a fork or spatula to make sure the walnuts are spread out and separated from one another while they cool. Otherwise they will clump together.

8   Once the walnuts have completely cooled, store them in an air-tight container. Enjoy as a nibble during work or study time, or toss them into a trail mix for a brain boost on the go!

DIY Sunflower Seed Butter

A plain old PB and J (or peanut butter and banana!) sandwich is one of my favorite brainiac snacks, and this sunflower seed butter is a treat on a sandwich. Pair it up with your favorite whole-grain or gluten-free bread. It's great on apple slices, too, and if you leave out the sugar I think it also pairs up nicely as a veggie dip with carrot sticks or celery.

Making sunflower seed butter at home is really easy, and the finished product tastes amazing. It's nice to switch things up in place of peanut butter for a change of pace, and if you can buy sunflower seeds in bulk from your local co-op or health food store it's also a really inexpensive option to make it yourself.

You can always use a store-bought seed or nut butter to make Sunpower Spread (see recipe in this chapter) if you are pressed for time, but you might enjoy making your own from scratch. All you need are some shelled sunflower seeds and a few minutes to work with a food processor.

Toasted seeds seem to work best for this, because the toasting process helps the seeds release their oils so they can blend better in your average food processor. Toasting also adds a nice roasty flavor to the finished sunflower butter that I really enjoy, and I think you will too!

How to Make

1   Spread the sunflower seeds onto a baking sheet with a rim and place them into a 350°F oven. It can take up to 20 minutes for them to toast properly, so keep an eye on them and stir every 10 minutes or so to get a feel for how they are doing. You want them to be golden brown and have a nutty smell.

2   Once the seeds are toasted, let them cool for 5–10 minutes, then transfer them to the bowl of a food processor. You will want the S-blade attachment on your food processor to make your seed butter.

3   Put the lid on the food processor and start grinding the seeds. It will take a little while before the butter starts to come together, perhaps as long as 5 minutes, so just be patient and go with it. I usually pulse for a few minutes and then turn it on while I work on other things. First, the seeds will grind down into a meal, and then the meal will start to become sticky and clump together. Keep processing, and after that the seeds will get to the butter stage.

4   Once the seeds have attained the perfect creamy, spreadable con-sistency, add sugar, salt, and coconut oil (if desired) and process another 1–2 minutes so that all the ingredients come together. If you are making Sunpower Spread, now is also the time to add 8 teaspoons (roughly $2\frac{1}{2}$ tablespoons) of Sunpower Powder.

5   Store the sunflower butter in an airtight container in the refrigera-tor until you are ready to use it. A serving of Sunpower Spread is 1–2 tablespoons. Enjoy as a spread on bread or crackers, or as a fruit or veggie dip.

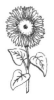

YIELDS APPROX.
2 CUPS

3 cups sunflower seeds
¼ cup (or to taste)
   sugar of your choice
   (optional)
Salt, to taste (optional)
2 tablespoons virgin
   coconut oil (optional)

Sunpower Powder and Spread

Sunflower seeds are a good source of choline, a micronutrient that is important during brain development and also appears to play a role in healthy memory and brain function as you age.

To make Sunpower Spread, you'll first need to make a batch of Sunpower Powder blend. You'll want to keep a batch of this Sunpower Powder on hand to easily add it to sunflower seed or nut butters whenever you want an extra dose of adaptogens to enhance your mental prowess. For this powder, mild-flavored ginkgo and rhodiola pair up with spicy rosemary for an adaptogen plus nootropic combination that's subtle and plays well with seed and nut butter. For each cup of Sunpower Spread that you want to mix up, you will need 4 teaspoons of this blend. That ratio will yield about ¼ teaspoon of herbal blend (1 serving) per tablespoon of Sunpower Spread.

Sunpower Powder

YIELDS 1 CUP (ENOUGH FOR 12 CUPS SUNPOWER SPREAD)

6 tablespoons powdered ginkgo leaves
4 tablespoons powdered rhodiola root
6 tablespoons powdered rosemary

How to Make

1 Place the powdered ginkgo, rhodiola, and rosemary into a medium mixing bowl and stir them gently until they are evenly combined.

2 When the herbs are blended together, transfer the powder to an airtight container, label the container, and store in a cool, dark place until you are ready to use.

Sunpower Spread

Stir in 4 teaspoons of powder per cup of sunflower seed butter until well blended, or add ¼-½ teaspoon of powder per serving in other recipes.

Food for Thought Chia Puddings

Chia seeds are a great source of protein and omega-3s, both of which are excellent ingredients for brain health. Plus, when you add liquid and allow them to gel they have a fun texture that makes a great, no-fuss pudding. Similar to flaxseed, chia seeds will "gel" with soluble fiber when exposed to liquids. Unlike flax, the seeds are barely noticeable in the finished gel, which makes chia a great option for breakfasts and snacks.

Three tablespoons of chia seeds usually sets up as a nice thick pudding in each of the following recipes, but if you find that your pudding is still a little thin, stir in another $\frac{1}{2}$ tablespoon and wait for 15 minutes to see how it sets up. If you add more chia seeds to these recipes, be sure not to skip that 15-minute rest. Eating chia before it gels can be uncomfortable—the seeds can start to expand when mixed with your saliva or the other liquids and be difficult to swallow as they keep expanding on the way down.

Chia pudding is the ultimate snack, dessert, or breakfast for busy people because it doesn't mind being thrown together in a hurry and then being left unsupervised overnight. Seriously—mix the ingredients together, let them sit in the refrigerator overnight so the chia seeds have a chance to gel, and you have a nutritious food ready when you wake up. Here are three super easy chia pudding recipes that include adaptogens.

All of these recipes make a single serving, but you can easily double or quadruple the recipe if you want to share or want to make ahead. You can even experiment with using different flavoring ingredients or other adaptogens besides the ones listed. My standard recipe formula for these is 3 tablespoons of chia seeds per 1 cup of liquid. If you already have a favorite chia pudding recipe, why not try adding your favorite adaptogen to the mix?

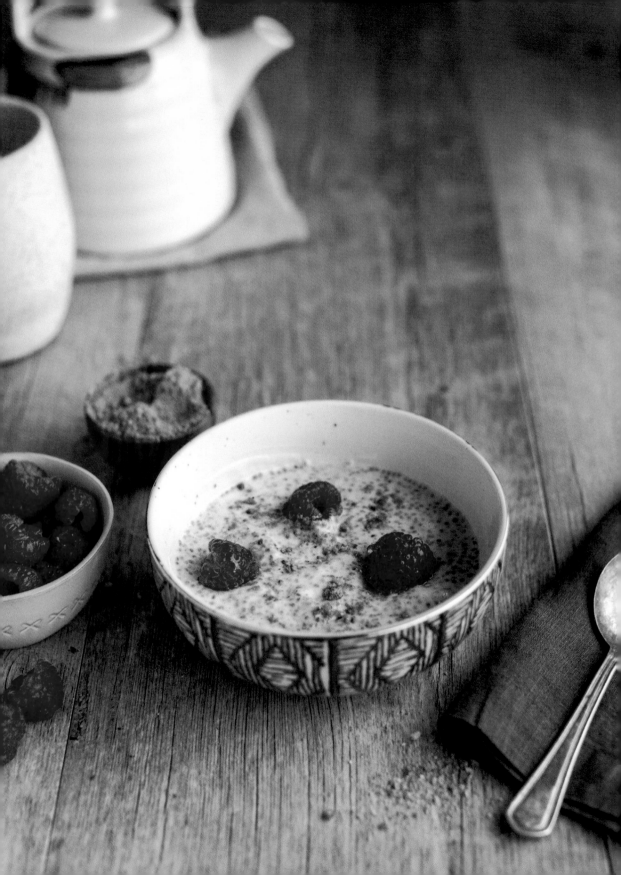

Raspberry and Rhodiola Chia Yogurt

Rhodiola is supportive for depressed mental states and helps you feel alert. It's been studied for its ability to enhance learning and improve memory, so that's why I chose it as the main ingredient for this recipe. I also just happen to like the taste of rhodiola and raspberries together!

Then again, I really like the taste of rhodiola even by itself. Its a little bit floral and is especially reminiscent of roses (hence its other name, roseroot). On its own, it's a little bitter, but not unpleasantly so. The taste of rhodiola isn't actually very noticeable in this particular recipe because the raspberries take center stage, but it is still there if you pay attention: just a hint of roses. And face it, raspberries are sassy and classy, and it's pretty hard to stay in a funk with something this fun in your mouth. So perk up and enjoy your Raspberry and Rhodiola Chia Yogurt!

How to Make

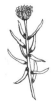

1 Whisk together the milk or plant milk, Greek yogurt, vanilla extract, rhodiola root powder, and sweetening syrup of your choice. Feel free to do this in a serving vessel if you are making a single serving. There's really no need to dirty an extra dish.

2 Whisk in the chia seeds.

3 Cover the bowl and put it in the refrigerator overnight.

4 In the morning, toss in a handful of fresh or frozen raspberries, top with some pistachios for crunch and extra protein, and enjoy!

YIELDS 1 SERVING

½ cup milk or vanilla-
    flavored plant milk
½ cup vanilla Greek yogurt
¼ teaspoon vanilla
    extract (optional)
¼ teaspoon powdered
    rhodiola root
1 tablespoon sweetening
    syrup of your choice:
    honey, agave, or
    maple syrup
3 tablespoons chia seeds
Raspberries (fresh if
    possible, but frozen
    berries also work)
Crushed pistachios, for
    garnish (optional)

Matcha and Peach Chia Seed Pudding with Gynostemma

I'm a Southern girl, so I love peaches, and I also love tea. My taste in tea has extended well beyond the regional fixation on sweet tea, though, so for this recipe you will find that matcha green tea pairs up delightfully well with fresh or frozen peaches and pecans for this chia bowl. Jiaogulan is mild, like nettles or green tea, so it won't compete with the matcha and peaches. Yum! You can also leave the fruit out for a more purely green tea experience. If you aren't feeling the Southern theme, try topping this bowl with shredded coconut, toasted buckwheat, or almond slivers instead of pecans.

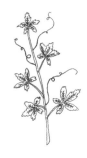

YIELDS 1 SERVING

1 cup milk or plant milk
2 teaspoons honey
½ teaspoon matcha
   powder
¼ teaspoon powdered
   jiaogulan
3 tablespoons chia
   seeds
Toppings: fresh or frozen
   peaches and pecan
   pieces

How to Make

1   In a cereal-sized bowl, whisk together the milk, honey, matcha powder, and jiaogulan powder. Add in the chia seeds and whisk until everything is combined.

2   Cover the bowl and allow it to rest in the refrigerator overnight.

3   Before serving this pudding, top it with peach slices and pecans, or other nutritional crunchies such as coconut, toasted buckwheat, or almond slivers.

Brainiac Oxymel

Oxymels have an unusual sweet-and-sour taste that comes from blending apple cider vinegar with honey. I often enjoy my oxymels as a flavoring for water by adding a few teaspoons to a glass of water and sipping on it. It's a fun way to add a little flavor and healthful benefits while you stay hydrated.

How to Make

1   Pour the vinegar into a glass jar and add the herbs and orange zest. Stir or shake everything (make sure to add the lid if you shake!) to combine all of the ingredients.

2   Pour the honey into the jar with the vinegar and herbs. Put the cap onto the jar, and give everything another good shake to dissolve the honey.

3   Label and date your oxymel. Store it in a dark place for 2–4 weeks, and give it a shake every day.

4   When the time is up and your oxymel is ready to use, you can either use it as is or strain the oxymel through a coffee filter to remove the powdered herbs.

5   To serve, add 1 teaspoon of the oxymel to 8 ounces of water. If you prefer, you can also dilute it in a 16-ounce glass of water. I prefer mine in cool water, but it's also good over ice.

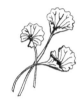

YIELDS ½ CUP
(24 SERVINGS)

¼ cup apple cider vinegar
1 tablespoon powdered gotu kola
½ tablespoon powdered ashwagandha
¼ teaspoon orange zest
¼ cup honey

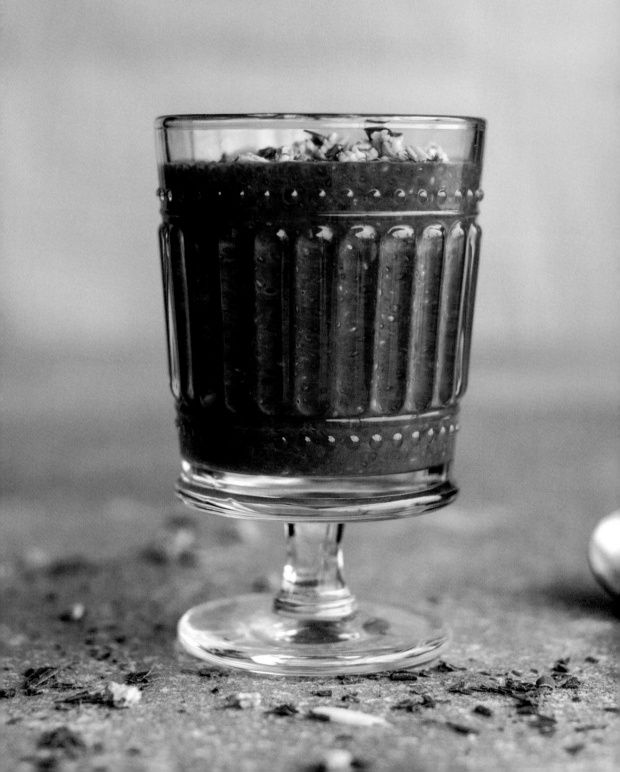

Ultimate Choco Chia Dessert Pudding

This chia pudding recipe is my excuse to eat chocolate for breakfast. Not that I really need an excuse (being an adult is pretty awesome), but it does make a nice incentive for eating breakfast on days when I'd really rather not. That's when the optional granola in the ingredient list comes in handy. Chia seeds are a good breakfast food, but granola definitely puts this on the list of valid and acceptable breakfast options. Usually, I'm only tempted to skip breakfast when I'm in a rush, so I make this the night before a busy day and grab it on my way out the door. When I'm feeling more like an adult and less like I need to bribe myself to eat breakfast, this recipe makes a nice less-guilt dessert option, sans granola.

The rich chocolaty flavor hides some of the less palatable adaptogens surprisingly well, so feel free to experiment with the adaptogens you prefer to support your mental prowess. Use ¼ teaspoon of powdered adaptogens total per serving.

How to Make

1 Whisk together the milk, cocoa powder, organic chocolate syrup, vanilla extract, salt, chia seeds, and shatavari powder in a serving bowl.

2 Place the pudding into the refrigerator overnight.

3 In the morning (or later in the day as a snack or dessert), add a handful of cacao nibs and granola to your pudding and enjoy!

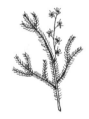

YIELDS 1 SERVING

1 cup milk or plant milk
1 tablespoon cocoa
  powder
2 tablespoons organic
  chocolate syrup
1 teaspoon vanilla
  extract
Dash sea salt (optional)
3 tablespoons chia
  seeds
¼ teaspoon shatavari
  powder
Cacao nibs and granola
  (optional)

Chili Lime Pistachios with Dang Shen (aka Dang Good Pistachios)

Dang shen, or codonopsis, is often described as being a milder alternative to ginseng. It has an overall mild and pleasant taste (I've heard that the fresh roots taste even better), and is ideal for gentle cognitive support. This recipe helps keep your brain food repertoire interesting with a zesty, spicy chili lime seasoning. These pistachios are good on their own or in trail mix, but they would also be really wonderful as a topping on a southwestern-themed salad.

Dang shen also has digestive system benefits and helps to improve digestion and the absorption of nutrients.

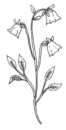

YIELDS 4 SERVINGS

1 cup shelled pistachios
2 teaspoons sesame oil
1 tablespoon honey
1 tablespoon lime juice
1 teaspoon garlic powder
⅛ teaspoon cayenne pepper (optional)
1 tablespoon sugar
1 teaspoon powdered dang shen
⅛ teaspoon sea salt

How to Make

1   Place the pistachios in a medium mixing bowl and set them aside. Preheat your oven to 350°F. You will also want to line a baking tray with parchment paper and keep it handy while you work.

2   Next, prepare the seasonings for the pistachios: combine the sesame oil, honey, lime juice, garlic powder, cayenne pepper, sugar, dang shen, and sea salt in a small saucepan over low heat. Stir gently until all of the ingredients have melted together.

3   Drizzle the mixture over the pistachios. Toss them gently to make sure they are evenly coated.

4   Spread the pistachios onto the lined baking tray, and bake them for around 20 minutes. Be sure to stir them at the 10-minute mark so they don't burn.

5   Remove the baking tray from the oven and allow the pistachios to cool. Store them in an airtight container.

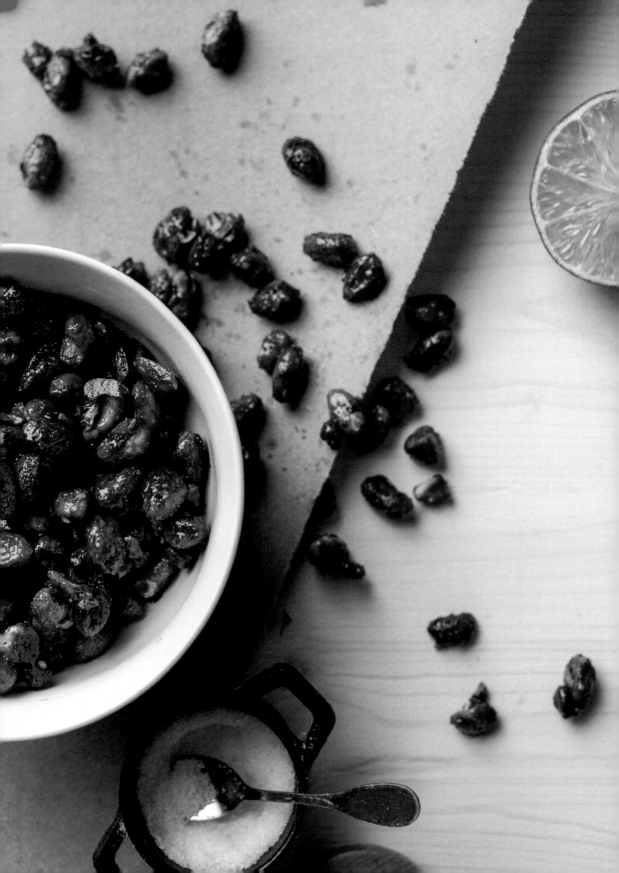

Brain Goo

When your brain feels like it's turning to mush from too much mental work or study, try some Brain Goo to get back in the groove. Rhodiola appears to support memorization and the ability to concentrate, and schisandra has your back with a simultaneous calming and focusing action. Add nootropics like gotu kola and ginkgo and you will be back to your books or projects with ease.

The technique for making a glycerite is very similar to that for making a vodka extract, but the end result is alcohol free, sweetish, and a bit gooey. Instead of using alcohol to extract the herbs, though, you will use a clear, viscous syrup called glycerin. Most of the time, you will need to add a little water to pre-moisten dried herbs when you make a glycerite so that the glycerin can do a better job as an extract. Otherwise the herbs will be too dry to extract well.

But what exactly is glycerin, besides a thick, clear syrup you can buy at the health food store? To understand glycerin, you need to know that most fats are triglycerides, which use glycerol and three fatty acids as their building blocks. Glycerin can be obtained by breaking down plant or animal fats. It's actually a byproduct of soap making, and commercial soap companies separate and distill the glycerin for resale.

Glycerin is sometimes used in foods and baked goods as a sweetener or to help keep foods moist because it is hygroscopic (meaning it attracts and holds moisture to the finished product to improve the texture and so that it doesn't dry out). Even though glycerin tastes sweet it doesn't raise blood sugar levels. In cosmetics, it's sometimes used as a humectant. You should make sure your glycerin is food grade if you are making an herbal glycerite.

The final product will be green and have a novel, slimy appeal…just kidding! It's actually only a little thicker than you might expect. A serving size is 60 drops, or about ½ teaspoon.

How to Make

1 Pour the glycerin and water into a 16-ounce jar and fasten the lid securely. Shake the jar until the glycerin and water are completely combined.

2 Add the powdered rhodiola root, schisandra berries, and gotu kola to the glycerin and water mixture.

3 Place the lid on the jar and shake it to combine the herbs and the liquid.

4 Let the glycerin and herbs macerate for 4 weeks. Give the jar a gentle shake every day.

5 At the end of 4 weeks, strain the herbs through a mesh sieve lined with a coffee filter or a jelly-making bag.

6 Bottle and label for use. Your glycerite should be shelf stable for 1–2 years.

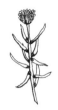

YIELDS APPROX.
3½ OUNCES
(40 SERVINGS)

3 ounces veggie glycerin
1 ounce water
2 teaspoons powdered
  rhodiola root
2 teaspoons powdered
  schisandra berries
2 teaspoons gotu kola

Thinking Cup

Personally, I like a little caffeine when I'm working on a project that requires my thinking cap, and thus was Thinking Cup created.

I find that coffee will make me jittery, but green tea has the perfect amount to help me focus and get the creative juices flowing. For reference, a cup of green tea can contain up to 70mg of caffeine, while a cup of coffee can have as much as 250mg of caffeine. Some people are more sensitive to the effects of caffeine. If you would prefer to go sans caffeine, you can leave out the green tea and use green rooibos instead. It tastes great with either.

If you like, quadruple the batch and keep it in a pitcher in the refrigerator to serve cold in the summer. Gotu kola and jiaogulan have mild flavors that go nicely with green tea, and make for a pleasant sip, warm or cold.

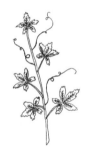

YIELDS 1 CUP
DRIED BLEND
(48 SERVINGS)

⅓ cup powdered
   jiaogulan
⅓ cup gotu kola
⅓ cup loose-leaf green
   tea or green rooibos

How to Make

1   Blend together the jiaogulan, gotu kola, and green tea or green rooibos, and store mixture in an airtight container in the pantry. Be sure to label it.

2   To make a tea, add 1 teaspoon of blend to a tea ball and place it in your favorite mug. Bring 1 cup of water to a boil, and pour the hot water into your cup.

3   Allow your tea to steep for 5–10 minutes, then remove the tea ball and sweeten your tea to taste.

Growing Jiaogulan

Jiaogulan makes a great houseplant or outdoor container plant. A cucurbit (related to the garden-variety cucumber, no less), this vine does best in part shade and is hardy down to about 20°F. It goes dormant in the winter, but you can expect a heavy harvest from a happy plant in the summer—it will send out plenty of tendrils in every direction! I have mine in a hanging basket and give it a home outside in the summer, but bring it indoors for winter. It doesn't like to dry out and needs a weekly meal of compost tea as a fertilizer to do best. To make a simple compost tea, add enough compost (preferably from your own compost pile, but a bag of store-bought compost will do in a pinch) to fill a 1-gallon bucket $\frac{1}{3}$ full. Add enough unchlorinated water to fill the bucket. Once a day for a week, stir the water and compost mixture. At the end of the week, your compost tea is ready and you can use it to water your jiaogulan! Your other container plants might appreciate it if you share it with them too.

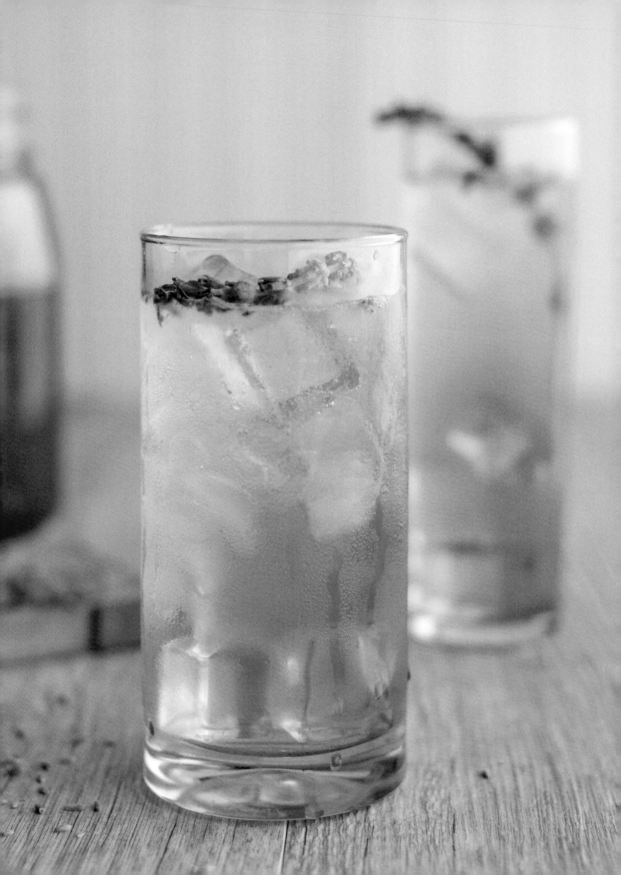

Lavender and Schisandra Syrup and Soda

With a little seltzer this easy syrup recipe makes an unusual lemony soda that's great when you are feeling too frazzled to concentrate. Lavender is a calming nervine, and schisandra is also calming to the nervous system. Schisandra supports focus and concentration, though, and with a bit of lemony zip to it, this soda won't put you to sleep.

I've fondly started calling this one my "study soda," and it's also been a hit when I have friends over and offer them some because I notice that they're feeling a bit stressed. It's refreshing and calming at the same time.

How to Make

1 Bring the water to a boil in a medium saucepan.

2 Add the schisandra berries to the boiling water and simmer over low heat for 20 minutes with the lid on. Turn off the heat and let the decoction steep for another 10 minutes.

3 Return the saucepan with the schisandra berries to the stovetop, and bring it to a boil once more. Turn off the heat once more and add the lavender buds. Let the herbs steep for an additional 3–5 minutes before straining.

4 Measure the liquid in a heat-safe measuring cup, and add more water if needed to bring it back to 1 cup of liquid.

5 Return the tea to the saucepan and add the sugar. Stir gently over low heat until the sugar has completely dissolved, and add the lemon juice.

6 Allow the syrup to cool, and store it in a glass canning jar in the refrigerator. It should be good for several weeks.

7 Stir 1–2 tablespoons of the Lavender and Schisandra Syrup into a glass of seltzer to create your schisandra soda. Add ice and garnish with a sprig of fresh lavender buds, if desired.

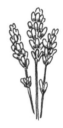

YIELDS 1½ CUPS SYRUP (12-24 SERVINGS)

16 ounces water
4 tablespoons dried schisandra berries
1 teaspoon lavender buds
1 cup sugar
Juice from 1 medium lemon (2–3 tablespoons)
1 sprig fresh lavender buds (optional)

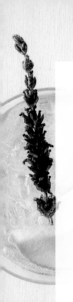

Combining Adaptogens

Most herbs play really well with other herbs, and adaptogens are no exception. Learning how to formulate herbs can include learning to make customized formulas for a certain individual based on his or her unique needs, as well as learning how to devise new formulas (or recipes!) meant to be used and enjoyed by many different people. Adaptogens combine very well with many other types of herbs, and even with each other. Many of the recipes in this book contain adaptogens plus other types of herbs, such as nervines or alteratives, or more than one kind of adaptogen. Even if you regularly take a certain adaptogen or have a particular favorite, it's fine to add other adaptogens or herbs to your routine.

Blackberry Brilliance Cordial

A cordial is made to be enjoyed in larger quantities than your typical elixir, so the herbal ingredient ratio is much lower but still high enough to be potent per serving size. This one is formulated so you can enjoy it either alone or as a mixed drink, so the serving size is 1.5 fluid ounces, rather than the usual drop measurements of an elixir or extract.

Impress your guests at your next dinner party, salon, or creative gathering, or share with a friend before you settle in for your next take-over-the-world brainstorming session. A toast to your brilliance!

How to Make

1 Combine the powdered eleuthero, rhodiola, white peony, rose petals, and chopped dried cherries with the brandy in a jar. Cap the jar with a lid.

2 Leave the cordial for 2–6 weeks to infuse. Give the jar a shake every day to help extract all of the goodness.

3 When the time is up, filter the herbs and fruit from the brandy. Add the honey or agave syrup, bottle it, and label the bottle. Enjoy your cordial the way you would any brandy, either neat or as a base for an inventive mixed drink.

YIELDS 21 SERVINGS

2 tablespoons eleuthero powder

2 tablespoons powdered rhodiola root

1 tablespoon white peony root powder

1 tablespoon dried rose petals

3 tablespoons chopped dried cherries

4 cups blackberry brandy

1 cup honey or agave nectar

Roasted Sweet Potatoes with Rosemary

Your brain uses glucose—sugar—for energy. Too much sugar can make you feel sleepy, but adding enough complex carbohydrates to your diet keeps your brain happy. Some good sources of complex carbs are corn, peas, lentils, and (as in this recipe) sweet potatoes. The complex carbs in sweet potatoes make for good brain food. This recipe doesn't call for many ingredients, but sometimes simple is better. These potatoes make a hearty, savory side dish or a snack. Add rosemary for flavor and brain health!

YIELDS 4 SERVINGS

4 medium sweet
    potatoes
2 tablespoons olive oil
Powdered rosemary,
    to taste
Salt and pepper, to taste

How to Make

1 Preheat the oven to 350°F.

2 Peel the sweet potatoes and cut them into bite-sized pieces.

3 Spread the sweet potato pieces onto a baking tray and drizzle them with olive oil.

4 Sprinkle rosemary onto the sweet potatoes and put them in the oven for 30 minutes. Check the sweet potato pieces with a fork—if they are soft all the way through they are ready.

5 Remove the tray from the oven and season the sweet potatoes with a little salt and pepper to taste.

Colorful Foods

Serving fruits and veggies in a variety of colors makes mealtime more interesting, and is also important for brain health. All of those colors are the results of flavonoids. Flavonoids help the ability of neurons to create and re-form connections with one another, a trait called synaptic plasticity. They also may help fight inflammation and give blood flow a healthy boost.

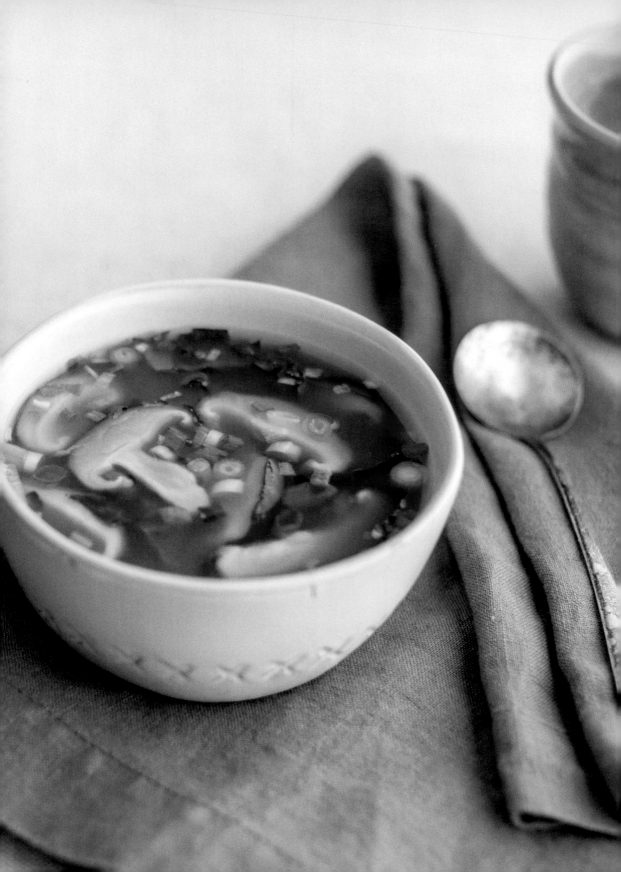

CHAPTER SIX

RECIPES TO IMPROVE YOUR IMMUNE FUNCTION

From what I've seen, immunity is a big deal for many people, and not just during the winter season when everyone is trying to fend off the sniffles, the ickies, and the latest stomach unhappiness. Immunity is really important during spring and fall allergy seasons too. Even summer can bring seasonal immunity issues from the occasional summer cold. And then there are always bigger immunity complications that we all want to do our best to avoid—autoimmune concerns and cancer being two of the biggest.

Herbalism is not a magic bullet for any of these immune challenges, but it does offer support to your body in ways that other modalities can't. Adaptogens are especially good at boosting stressed-out immune systems and promoting healthy immune function, often helping to bring balance to overactive and underactive immune systems alike.

Although all adaptogens have an effect on the immune system to some extent, certain adaptogens are considered to have an overall normalizing effect on the immune system. Herbs like reishi, schisandra, licorice, ashwagandha, cordyceps, and the ginsengs fall into this category.

Other adaptogens have somewhat more specific immune uses. Licorice, holy basil, and reishi have made reputations for themselves when it comes to immune systems on the defensive and preoccupied with allergens. Eleuthero and rhodiola seem to be able to protect immunity from dipping in athletes under heavy training regimens. Astragalus has developed a reputation for being the go-to adaptogen when immunity and overall health seem to be run down.

Burdock is an adaptogen that also has alterative properties. Alteratives are herbs that seem to be especially good at helping the body with the elimination of wastes and acting as a metabolic tonic. In this capacity, it helps the lymphatic system function at its best just as much as it helps the liver, kidneys, and digestive and endocrine systems.

Besides herbs that support a healthy immune system, people seem to be especially interested in herbs that can be used instead of antibiotics. Chances are, that laundry list of "antibiotic" herbs you printed from the Internet is mostly incorrect. There are a lot of herbs that get tossed around in this category just because they contain one or two ingredients that can potentially have antimicrobial properties. Unfortunately, even though an herb has an ingredient that might be antimicrobial alone and in sufficient quantities in a laboratory setting, that doesn't mean it will behave that way in the human body. Herbalism largely focuses on supporting a healthy immune system because that's what herbs do best!

The recipes in this chapter cover a number of different ways to add immune-supportive adaptogens to your diet that go beyond taking capsules or relying on an extract. Of course there's nothing wrong with capsules or extracts, but these recipes are meant to take things a little further by adding extra nutrition and interest to your immune-supportive routines. Let's face it—it's easier to remember to take something yummy that you look forward to and enjoy! Trying to remember to swallow a pill 3 times a day or finding a way to chase a less-than-appetizing extract is no fun.

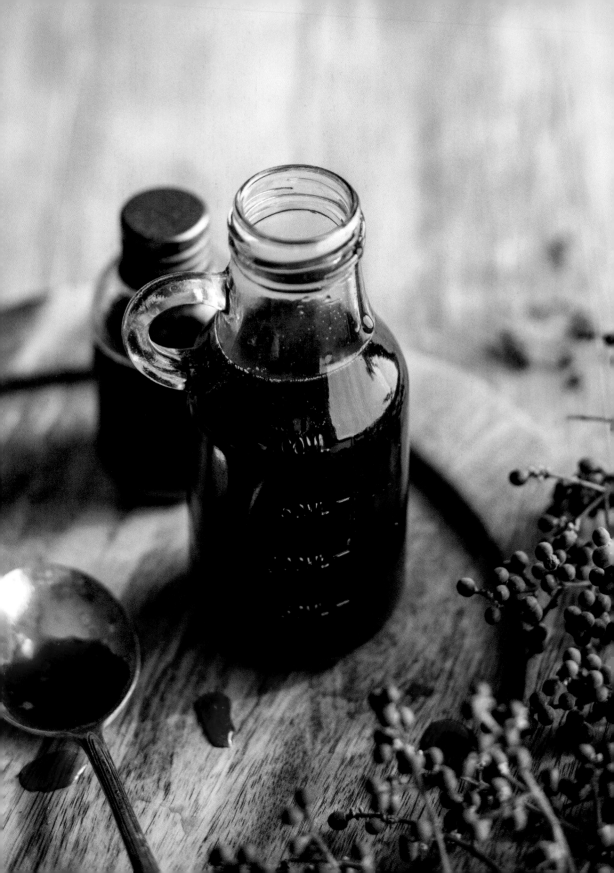

Goji and Elderberry Syrup

You're probably familiar with elderberry syrup. It's extremely popular in health-conscious circles during wintertime, and for good reason. Elderberry tastes good and it has plenty of studies to back it up as an immune stimulant that increases cytokine production and also may help to strengthen cell walls to prevent viruses from entering. Making your own syrup is fun and inexpensive, and lets you customize it with your favorite flavorings and add awesome adaptogenic ingredients to the brew!

Because this syrup contains astragalus, it's great if you are trying to stay well, but not so great if you are starting to feel sick. Traditionally speaking, astragalus should not be used during acute illness, so discontinue it and switch to a plain elderberry syrup if you start to feel under the weather, and go see your doctor if you need to.

A serving of Goji and Elderberry Syrup is 1 tablespoon. You can take it all at once or split it into 3 teaspoons over the course of the day.

How to Make

1   Place the elderberries, goji berries, rose hips, astragalus root, and licorice root in a small saucepan with 16 ounces of water.

2   Simmer the herbs over low heat with the lid on until the water has reduced to 8 ounces. Usually this will take around 20 minutes. Leave the herbs in the decoction and allow it to steep in the refrigerator overnight. (If you are in a hurry, you can skip this step, but allowing it to steep overnight makes the finished syrup more concentrated.)

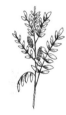

YIELDS 8 OUNCES

¼ cup dried elderberries
1 tablespoon dried goji berries
1 tablespoon rose hips
2 tablespoons cut and sifted astragalus root
1 teaspoon cut and sifted licorice root
16 ounces water
8 ounces honey

3   Strain the herbs through a sieve and double-check that you have 8 ounces of brew after all the herbs have been removed.

4   Place the decoction back into the saucepan and add the honey. Warm the brew over low heat just until the honey has combined with the decoction.

5   Once the honey has dissolved, immediately remove the syrup from the heat. At this point you can leave it as is and store the syrup in the refrigerator, or if you want a shelf-stable syrup you can add 5 ounces of brandy or vodka to the syrup.

Adaptogens for Children

Some adaptogens, like astragalus, are commonly
used for children. Other adaptogens may be too
strong or too stimulating for young children.
There's not a lot of safety data available on using
adaptogens for children. A child's metabolism is
somewhat different than an adult's, so if you are
considering the use of adaptogens for younger
members of your household, be sure to check
in with an herbalist and your pediatrician to get
their opinions.

Astragalus Multi-Grain Bowls

Astragalus and mushrooms beg to be added to soups and stock. On its own, astragalus has a taste that is bland and a little bitter. It reminds me of the way pencil shavings smell. Add a few other savory ingredients and seasonings, though, and you can mask the taste of the astragalus in the finished recipe. I find that mushrooms and garden sage are generally up to the task.

You can use any combination of grains that you like, so feel free to experiment. Just make sure to use 1 cup of brown rice and 1 cup of mixed grains to keep the ratio correct.

How to Make

1　Make a decoction with the astragalus root by simmering it in a small saucepan over low heat for 20 minutes in the broth and then straining.

2　If using quinoa, prewash your mixed grains to remove any bitter saponins from the outside of the quinoa.

3　Measure out 3 cups of broth/decoction, and pour it into a large bowl with your grains. Add a little water or extra broth if you need to so that you have 3 cups of liquid. Place the mixed grains and rice in the refrigerator overnight to presoak.

4　In the morning, put the grains, the seaweed seasoning blend, and the decoction into a rice cooker and start the cooking process as usual. Use the brown rice setting for best results.

5　If you are using a stovetop method, place the grains and decoction into a saucepan and bring to a simmer over low heat. Simmer for 30 minutes, then cover, remove from the heat, and allow it to steam with the lid on for 10 minutes.

6　Add salt to taste before serving. Serve with sautéed shiitakes, garlic, and veggies of your choice.

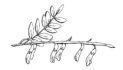

YIELDS 4 SERVINGS

2 tablespoons cut and
　sifted astragalus root
3½ cups broth of your
　choice
1 cup mixed grains
　(quinoa, amaranth,
　millet, and so on)
1 cup brown rice
1 teaspoon seaweed
　seasoning blend
Salt, to taste

Amla and Ginger Instant Tea

Licorice and ginger is a good combo to remember during allergy season. Ginger has a warming, drying action on the upper respiratory tract, and licorice helps support your immune system. Amla has immune-supporting properties of its own, and also has a yummy flavor.

Use powdered herbs for the easiest tea—just stir it all up and enjoy your drink!

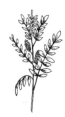

YIELDS 24 SERVINGS

1 tablespoon powdered
   licorice root
4 tablespoons powdered
   amla berries
3 tablespoons ground
   ginger
8 ounces water

How to Make

1   Blend together the powdered licorice root, amla berries, and ginger and store them in an airtight container. Make sure to label your tea so you can find it easily when you need it.

2   To make a cup of tea, bring 8 ounces of water to a boil and add 1 teaspoon of amla and ginger blend. Allow to simmer for 10 minutes.

3   Pour into your favorite mug. The licorice and goji have a sweet taste, so be sure to take a sip before you reach for your favorite sweetener. You may not need it.

4   If you are in a hurry, you can boil 8 ounces of water and pour it into a thermos. Add 1 teaspoon of Amla and Ginger Instant Tea, and allow it to steep with the thermos lid on for 10 minutes before you drink it. Simmering as per step 2 helps the herbs release their goodness, but since you are working with a powder and drinking it down rather than straining it out at the end, it's not as necessary to use a standard decocting process.

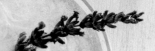

Adaptogens for the Compost

When you make an herbal tea or an extract, you can save the used up herbs and put them into your compost heap or sprinkle them around your garden on top of the soil. Your plants will love them. As a general rule, fats and oils don't belong in the compost pile, but even if your herbs are from a project made with an oil infusion you may still find that they won't do any harm. As long as you blend the oil-soaked herbs well with the other compost materials, they should be all right. Don't pour rancid infused oils onto the compost heap, however. That much oil can definitely interfere with the composting process.

Burdock Skillet Sauté

This is a casual skillet meal that plays on the popular combination of carrots and burdock as stir-fry ingredients. Burdock root is a little bit earthy but pairs really well with carrots, kale, and shiitake mushrooms in the simplicity of a one-pan vegetarian meal or a yummy side dish. I like to sauté the burdock and carrot somewhat briefly so that there is plenty of crunch left in the final dish.

For this recipe, use a guillotine slicer or veggie peeler to get paper-thin pieces of the roots. Leaving peels on will make the finished dish a little less sweet and make the burdock's earthiness more pronounced. You might want to peel the burdock and carrots the first time you make this.

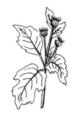

YIELDS 2–4 SERVINGS

3 tablespoons diced shiitake mushrooms
1 clove garlic, peeled and finely chopped
1 tablespoon sesame oil
1 cup very thin carrot slices
1 cup very thin burdock root slices
2 cups kale leaves, cut into strips
2 tablespoons water
1 tablespoon tamari

How to Make

1 In a medium skillet, sauté the mushrooms and garlic in the sesame oil over medium heat until they are soft (usually around 5 minutes). Add the carrot and burdock slices and sauté for a few minutes until they just begin to soften.

2 Add the kale and the water, and apply a cover or lid so that the kale can steam quickly.

3 When the kale softens after 2–3 minutes, remove the lid and stir as the water evaporates.

4 Add the tamari, stir to combine, and serve as a side dish or over rice.

Run Ragged Extract

I like the berry flavor of amla in this easy extract. It pairs up for a tasty blend with plain old eleuthero. If you feel like your immunity has taken a hit thanks to a higher than usual load of stress, this one might be a good option for you.

Eleuthero can help protect the immune systems of athletes during intense training. After a certain point during physical training, the immune system can really begin to struggle. It's a perfect example of how too much of a good thing (exercise) can actually be a bad thing. Still, we often strive for that new personal record, or wonder just how far we can push and stretch and how much we can achieve. If you're going to put yourself through the wringer, the least you can do is give yourself a little extra support.

Sometimes, of course, life puts us through the wringer whether we want to be there or not. It's nice to have options to support our best health, no matter what we are working through!

How to Make

1 Mix the powdered amla berries and powdered eleuthero together in a jar.

2 If you wish to make a percolation extract, follow the directions for the project "Make an Herbal Extract by Percolation" in Chapter 1. If you are making a regular maceration extract, pour the 5 ounces of vodka into the jar, cap it with a lid, and give everything a good shake to combine.

3 Allow your extract to macerate for 2–4 weeks. Check on it every day and give it a shake. You should see at least an inch of vodka covering the herbs before you shake the jar. Add a little extra vodka if needed to keep the herbs covered. After the 2–4 weeks are up, strain and bottle your extract. As with all alcohol-based extracts, your Run Ragged Extract should be shelf stable at room temperature for several years. A good serving size for this extract is 30 drops up to 3 times a day.

YIELDS AROUND 3½–4 OUNCES

½ ounce amla berry powder
½ ounce eleuthero powder
5 ounces vodka (plus a little extra if you're planning to make a percolation extract)

Strawberry Eleuthero Shrub

Shrubs, also known as drinking vinegars, are an interesting take on the vinegar-based extract for the savvy herbalist. Shrubs were a big thing in colonial America as a way to preserve and enjoy fruit without refrigeration, but eventually they fell out of popularity. Modern foodies and tipplers have brought them back because the sweet-and-sour profile is lots of fun, and there is plenty of room to let your creativity shine by orchestrating unique combinations of fruits, vinegars, and spices.

You will need two components for the shrub: a vinegar herbal extract and a fruit syrup. The vinegar will take the longest amount of time to prepare, so make sure it's ready before you proceed to making the fruit syrup. You will need to let your herbal vinegar steep for a few weeks before turning it into a shrub.

The method presented here for making the fruit syrup is a very traditional cold-process way. Some people prefer a stovetop method, but I like being able to stir it together and let it do its thing while I'm busy elsewhere. Also, the flavors are brighter using the cold-press method, which is an extra bonus! You can always make the syrup when the strawberries are in season and freeze it for later. That way you can make a batch of Strawberry Eleuthero Shrub when you want an immune boost the most.

Eleuthero Vinegar Extract

YIELDS 2 CUPS

2 ounces eleuthero powder
2 cups apple cider vinegar

How to Make

1 Combine the eleuthero and the vinegar in a glass jar. Label your jar so you don't forget what's inside, and let your herbs and vinegar sit for a minimum of 2 weeks.

2 After 2-4 weeks, your vinegar will be ready to strain and you can begin to make your syrup. If you want, you can wait to strain the vinegar until the syrup is ready or you can strain the vinegar and set it aside in a clean glass canning jar with a lid until it is time to combine it with the syrup.

Shrub Fruit Syrup

YIELD WILL VARY BASED ON JUICE CONTENT OF THE STRAWBERRIES

2 cups chopped fresh strawberries
2 cups sugar

How to Make

1 Place the chopped strawberries in a medium bowl, and toss them with the sugar until all the berry pieces are nicely coated.

2 Cover the bowl and place it in the refrigerator for 1-2 days, until the berries have released lots of juice.

3 Strain out the fruit, and reserve the liquid and any leftover sugar that may have settled on the bottom of the bowl. Now you are ready to make the shrub!

Strawberry Eleuthero Shrub

YIELDS 4 CUPS

2 cups Shrub Fruit Syrup (with leftover sugar)
2 cups Eleuthero Vinegar Extract

How to Make

1   In a medium mixing bowl, combine the Shrub Fruit Syrup, along with any leftover sugar that has yet to dissolve, and the Eleuthero Vinegar Extract.

2   Bottle and label your shrub in a single jar or bottle. Resist the urge to bottle in smaller bottles, at least at first. The vinegar will dissolve the remaining sugar.

3   The shrub's flavor profile will change over time as the vinegar goes to work on the sugars in the syrup. Eventually it may completely change into a fruit vinegar, so store it in the refrigerator and use it within 1–2 months for best results.

4   To make a serving of Strawberry Eleuthero Shrub, use 1–2 tablespoons and mix it into still or sparkling water, or use it in a cocktail recipe.

More Adaptogens Plz! Miso

I love a savory cup of miso soup for any occasion, but it's a particular favorite if I'm feeling under the weather. In case you are uninitiated to the cult of miso, let's take a peek at the different styles of miso paste that are available at your local health food store or international farmers' market. Miso is a paste made from fermented soybeans and grains and is part of Chinese and Japanese cuisine. It comes in different colors. White miso is the mildest and sweetest, followed by yellow miso and red miso with stronger, saltier flavors.

Although I'm not typically a fan of soy in its raw, unfermented form (as it is so often used in the Western diet), fermenting seems to take the edge off the phytic acids in soy that can interfere with nutrient absorption. Fermented foods are also a good way to introduce probiotics into the diet, so go with an unpasteurized miso paste if you can find one! Miso is sometimes made with gluten-containing grains such as barley, but it can also be made with rice. Be sure to read labels if you need a gluten-free option.

Here's a basic miso soup recipe that includes some immune system–fortifying adaptogens in the broth. Dashi (a traditional Japanese broth made with kombu seaweed and bonito fish flakes) is an even more traditional option than the water or veggie broth, but any of the three makes a very nice miso.

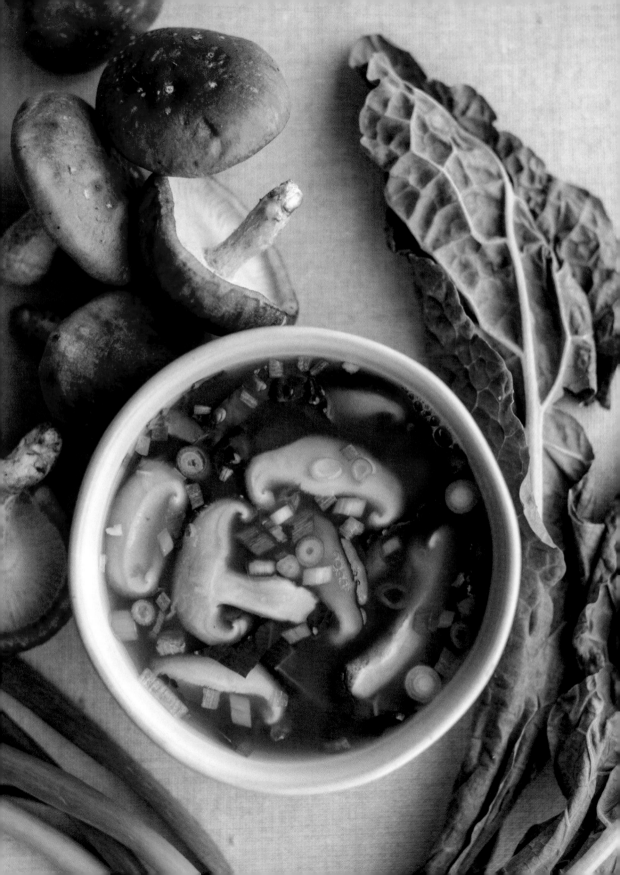

How to Make

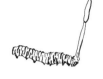

YIELDS 1 (1-CUP)
SERVING

1½ cups water or
vegetable broth
¼ teaspoon cordyceps
powder
¼ teaspoon astragalus
root powder
2 tablespoons chopped
shiitake mushrooms
2 tablespoons white
miso paste, or to taste
1 cup thinly sliced kale
1 tablespoon chopped
green onions
(optional)

1   In a small saucepan, combine the water or broth, cordyceps powder, and astragalus root powder. Simmer for 20 minutes over low heat, allow to cool, and strain through a coffee filter to remove the herbs.

2   Measure to make sure you have 1 cup of remaining liquid, and add extra if needed.

3   Return the decoction to the saucepan over low heat and bring it up to a simmer. Add the shiitake mushrooms.

4   Put 2 tablespoons of miso paste into a serving bowl while the mushrooms simmer. Take a few tablespoons of the simmering decoction and add it to the miso paste. Add the kale to the saucepan. While the kale and mushrooms continue to cook, gently stir the miso paste and liquid to thin the miso paste.

5   When the kale and mushrooms are cooked to your liking, pour your decoction into the serving bowl and stir gently until the miso liquid is mixed in.

6   Garnish with the chopped green onions and serve.

Chicken Noodle Soup with—Miso?

The next time you make yourself a comforting bowl of chicken soup, consider adding a dab of white miso paste. It adds a delicious accent to typical chicken soup (noodles, carrots, chicken, and a little onion, garlic, and parsley). Try this tasty East meets West soup when you need something a little extra-nourishing to get you through the day.

Immune Berry Astragalus Gummies

Have you seen gummy vitamins on the shelf at your local health food store? Originally they were just for kids, but more and more companies are making them for the adult crowd too. These astragalus gummies are better tasting than any of the ones from the store, and contain fewer preservatives (that is, none). Here's another plus: the only sweetness comes from the fruit itself!

You shouldn't devour these at quite the same rate as your favorite gummy bear candies, but you can use 3–6 gummies per day. If you have any liquid left over, you can add an equal amount of honey to make a syrup and enjoy it a few teaspoons at a time.

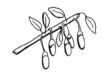

YIELDS 75 (1")
GUMMIES

3 cups cherry, purple grape, or pomegranate juice
½ cup dried elderberries
¼ cup cut and sifted astragalus root
2 tablespoons amla berries
2 tablespoons goji berries
½ cup plain, unflavored gelatin powder

How to Make

1 Simmer the juice, elderberries, astragalus root, amla berries, and goji berries in a medium saucepan over low heat for 20 minutes.

2 Remove the mixture from the heat and strain it into a heat-safe measuring cup.

3 Measure out 2 separate cups of the liquid. One cup should go into a heat-safe bowl and sit in the refrigerator until cold. The other cup of liquid can go back into the saucepan.

4 Once the juice in the refrigerator is cold, sprinkle the gelatin on top and let it rest for a few minutes. This allows the gelatin to "bloom," or reconstitute, before the next step.

5 Bring the cup of juice in the saucepan to a simmer, and then pour it over the cold juice and gelatin mixture.

6 Stir the gelatin and juice together briskly with a whisk until the gelatin is completely dissolved. From there, use a dropper to transfer the liquid from the saucepan into silicone candy molds. If you don't have candy molds, you can pour the liquid into a glass baking pan.

7 Stash the filled candy molds (or glass baking pan) in the refrigerator for 1–2 hours to cool and harden, then remove the gummies from the candy molds (if using the glass baking pan, cut the gelatin into 1"-2" cubes) and store in an airtight container in the fridge.

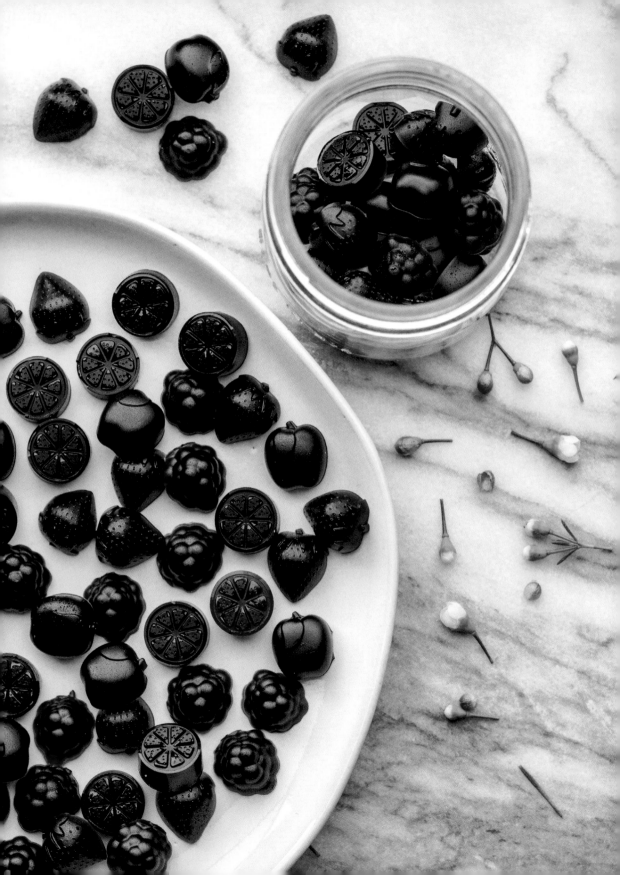

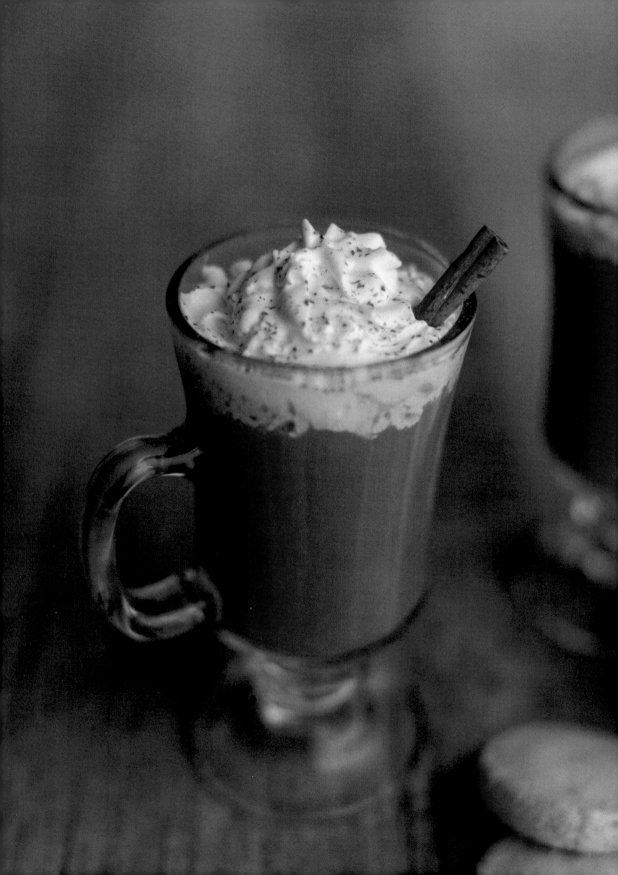

Cinnamon Cordyceps Cocoa

Mushrooms go surprisingly well with chocolate in terms of taste. Let's face it, though—most things go pretty well with chocolate! Medicinal fungi like chaga, reishi, and cordyceps are typical candidates for mushroom hot cocoa. Many recipes call for making a tea with the mushrooms and using that as a base, which can be a lot of work for a simple cup of cocoa. A creamier cocoa has no problem carrying ¼ teaspoon of cordyceps powder, though, so I like to make mine the easy way outlined here.

Word to the wise: make sure your cordyceps are from a cultivated source. Not only are wild cordyceps a parasite on dead caterpillars…well, they're a parasite on dead caterpillars. This leaves something to be desired in terms of potential bacterial contamination and also in mental imagery. The fungus invades a living caterpillar and kills it, then the spores fruit from the remains. (It makes you wonder if the first person to try cordyceps took a good look at where it was growing.)

There's also an issue of overharvesting in their native habitat. Everything has a purpose when in balance, so let's leave the wild cordyceps to do their thing. Cultivated cordyceps are grown on soybeans and/or grains. That's a bit more appetizing to reflect upon while you enjoy your cocoa!

How to Make

1 Warm up 6 ounces of milk or nut milk in a small saucepan over medium-high heat.

2 Stir in 2 tablespoons of organic hot cocoa mix and ¼ teaspoon cordyceps powder. Stir in a bit of butter or cream, if desired.

3 Pour your cocoa into a mug. Top with whipped cream if desired and sprinkle cinnamon on top. Garnish with a cinnamon stick if desired.

YIELDS 1 (1-CUP) SERVING

6 ounces milk or nut milk
2 tablespoons organic hot cocoa mix (or follow the directions on your blend)
¼ teaspoon cordyceps powder
Dash of cream or bit of butter (if you're feeling extra decadent)
Whipped cream to top (optional)
Ground cinnamon, to taste
Cinnamon stick, for garnish (optional)

Maple Ginger Immune Elixir

Maple, ginger, and vanilla make this immune elixir really fun and different than the typical immune flavor options of elderberry, more elderberry, and extra elderberry... and sometimes chocolate. Not that I have anything against elderberry or chocolate, but a change is definitely nice.

Dang shen, also known as codonopsis, is a gentle immune tonic. Holy basil is classified as an immunomodulator or amphoteric—an herb that helps bring balance to the immune system. In *Adaptogens: Herbs for Strength, Stamina, and Stress Relief*, herbalist David Winston notes that he frequently uses holy basil for clients who are dealing with allergies, so don't feel that you have to limit this elixir to your winter wellness repertoire.

To make your elixir, you will need holy basil and codonopsis extracts. I run both of mine through the percolation process at the same time, but you can choose to make them with a basic maceration process if you prefer. The ingredients listed here should yield around 4 ounces.

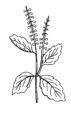

YIELDS 4 OUNCES (30–60 DROPS)

2 ounces codonopsis
   extract
2 ounces holy basil
   extract
2 ounces maple syrup
1" piece peeled fresh
   gingerroot
½ vanilla bean

How to Make

1 Combine 2 ounces of each extract in a glass jar to make a blend for the elixir.

2 Add maple syrup, fresh ginger, and ½ vanilla bean to the jar and allow to sit in a cool, dark place for at least 1 week before using so that the flavors meld. You can leave the vanilla and ginger in the jar, or remove them when you are happy with the taste.

Why a Cool, Dark Place?

Most of my extract and elixir recipes will tell you to store your herbal preparations in a cool, dark place. You may be wondering just how important it is to follow this suggestion. Herbs contain a complex array of compounds and naturally occurring chemical ingredients: alkaloids, polysaccharides, flavonoids, and volatile oils, just to name a few! Most of these ingredients are sensitive to heat and direct light and will degrade more quickly when exposed. Moisture is another important consideration, especially for dried herbs. Plant material will easily begin to mold if it gets damp. That's why it's best to store your dried herbs in airtight containers and keep them away from damp places in your home, such as basements and bathrooms.

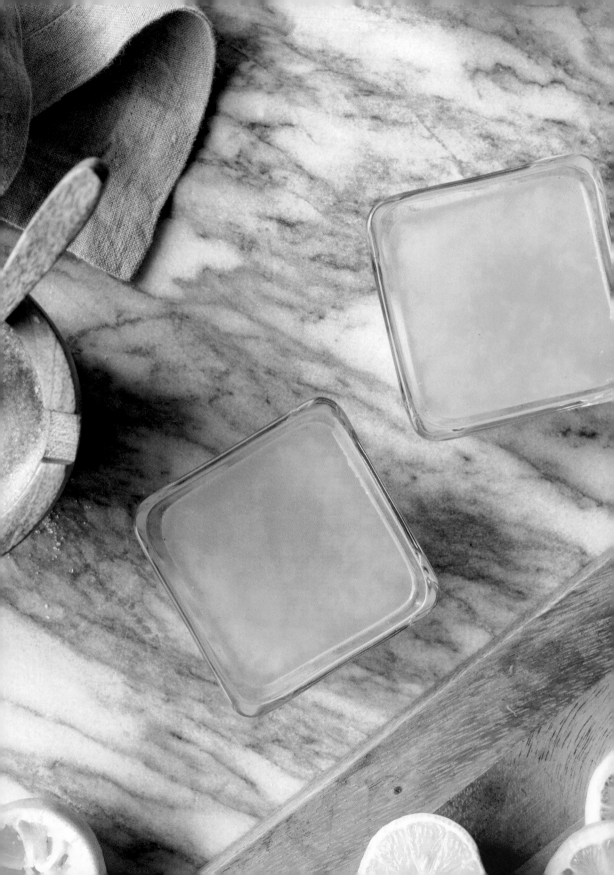

CHAPTER SEVEN

RECIPES TO IMPROVE YOUR ENERGY AND STAMINA

Eleuthero, rhodiola, and ginseng are some of the most popular adaptogens to improve energy and stamina. Whether you work in a physically demanding job, are an extreme sports enthusiast, or simply want to boost your general daily energy levels, adaptogens can offer support!

Pay attention to the time of day when you consistently feel a dip in your energy levels. According to traditional Chinese herbalism, each 2-hour increment during the day is "governed" by a different organ system. If you notice a consistent pattern, talk with an herbalist. That system may be in need of a tune-up!

What else makes a big difference in our daytime energy levels? Sleep! I know, nobody likes to sleep when there is so much living to be done, but your body needs it. And if you're like most people I observe and talk to, you don't get enough of it. Unplug, turn off the bright screens well before bedtime, and develop an evening routine that helps your body find a natural rhythm. Your daytime self will thank you with better concentration, energy, and alertness with which to fully enjoy all of that crazy living.

Although this chapter is all about energy and stamina, let's take a quick look at herbs that support that all-important healthy night of sleep. A certain classification of herbs known as nervines are especially adept at this task. Herbs can belong to more than one category, and holy basil and ashwagandha are perfect examples. Both are adaptogens with nervine properties. Nervines behave in ways that are very complementary to the actions of adaptogens—namely, they nourish the nervous system and help promote a healthy response to stress. Some nervines are good for daytime use—linden and passionflower are two that come to mind here—while others, like hops, are more commonly associated with evening use. For a few great night owl recipes to help put your inner roadrunner to bed, be sure to read through Chapter 4: Recipes to Improve Your Mood.

24-Hour Qi Cycle

Curious about which organ systems correspond to which times of day? This is a Chinese herbalism concept that describes how energy flows from one system to another over the course of the day. At a certain point every 24 hours, an organ system is believed to be at its most optimal time of functioning. Here's a quick glimpse into this body clock:

- 1:00 a.m.—3:00 a.m.   Liver

- 3:00 a.m.—5:00 a.m.   Lung

- 5:00 a.m.—7:00 a.m.   Large intestine

- 7:00 a.m.—9:00 a.m.   Stomach

- 9:00 a.m.—11:00 a.m.   Spleen

- 11:00 a.m.—1:00 p.m.   Heart

- 1:00 p.m.—3:00 p.m.   Small intestine

- 3:00 p.m.—5:00 p.m.   Bladder

- 5:00 p.m.—7:00 p.m.   Kidney

- 7:00 p.m.—9:00 p.m.   Pericardium

- 9:00 p.m.—11:00 p.m.   Triple burner/Blood vessels and arteries

- 11:00 p.m.—1:00 a.m.   Gallbladder

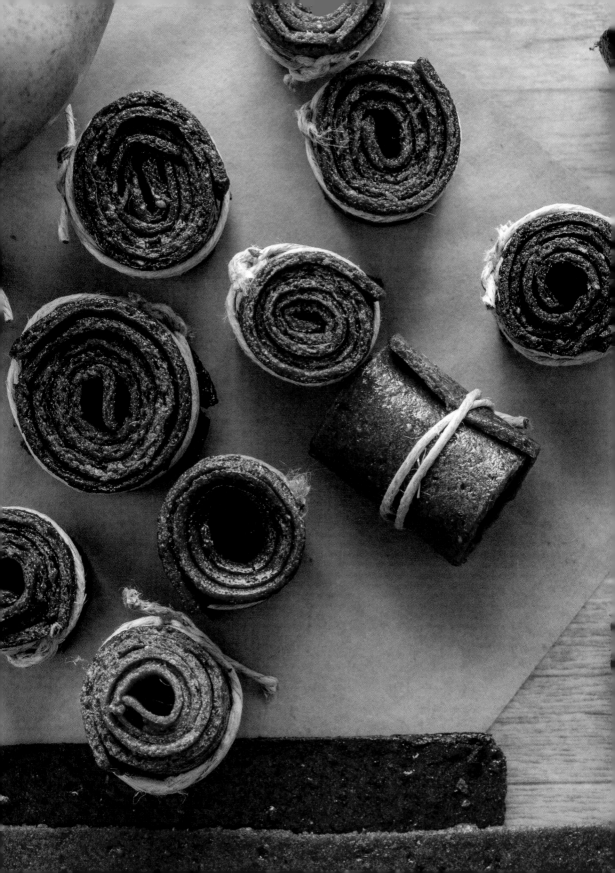

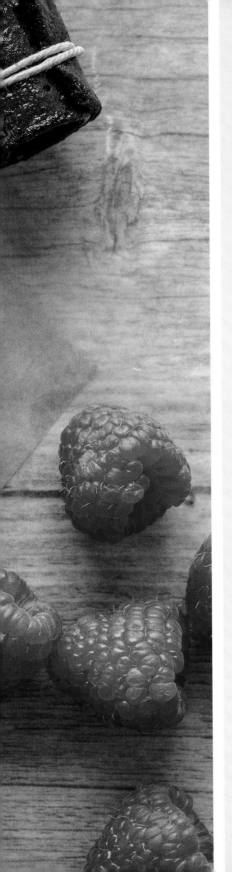

Rhodiola Fruit Leathers

Remember fruit roll-ups when you were a kid? I bet you can remember (with appropriate shame) your love for bright red, artificially flavored sheets of sugar paste. It's okay, I don't think I've ever met a kid (myself included!) who didn't have an unholy fascination with this sweet concoction. But move over, nostalgia. It's time for something even better to nosh.

The next step up from the fruit roll-up is fruit leather. These are made with actual fruit, and are sort of like fruit jerky—thick, chewy, and pretty satisfying. The following recipes use applesauce to make the finished fruit leather more flexible, and you don't have to worry about pre-cooking the fruit. You can use a dehydrator for these or dry them in the oven at 200°F on a 9" × 13" baking pan for about 6 hours. Prepare the pans with baking spray or a nonstick silicone baking mat to make it easy to remove the leather when it's ready.

Which adaptogen extracts should you use? Personally, I like the way rhodiola blends with just about any fruit, but you can switch things up and use whatever you like. Rather than use powders for these recipes I've chosen to add the liquid extracts. The powders would probably work just as well, though; you would need about ¼ teaspoon of finely ground powder per serving if you want to experiment.

The recipes call for frozen berries, but you can use fresh if they are available. Choose one of these three recipes to get your fruit leather fix:

Pear Blueberry Fruit Leathers

YIELDS 9 SERVINGS

1 cup pureed soft, ripe pears
½ cup pureed frozen blueberries
½ cup applesauce
¼ cup honey
2 teaspoons lemon juice
3–6 teaspoons adaptogen extract(s)

Cherry Raspberry Fruit Leathers

YIELDS 9 SERVINGS

1 cup pureed frozen cherries
½ cup pureed frozen raspberries
½ cup applesauce
¼ cup honey
2 teaspoons lemon juice
3–6 teaspoons adaptogen extract(s)

Simply Strawberry Fruit Leathers

YIELDS 9 SERVINGS

1½ cups pureed strawberries
½ cup applesauce
¼ cup honey
2 teaspoons lemon juice
3–6 teaspoons adaptogen extract(s)

How to Make

1 Preheat your oven to 200°F. Combine the pureed fruit, honey, lemon juice, and adaptogen extract(s) in a medium bowl and mix well.

2 Spread the fruit mixture onto a baking pan that has been prepped with a silicone baking mat or baking spray. Make sure the baking pan has a rim to stop the ingredients from sliding off during the drying process, but try to keep the fruit leather mixture toward the middle of the pan for more even drying. A 9" × 13" pan should give you plenty of room.

3 Bake your fruit leather for 6 hours with the oven door open a little. Check the fruit leather every few hours to make sure it doesn't brown. You want it to be dry to the touch, which should happen somewhere around the 6-hour mark.

4 When the fruit leather is dry to the touch, turn off the oven and close the oven door. Leave the fruit leather overnight to continue the drying process.

5 Cut the fruit leather into 9 even strips the next day. Roll up each strip on a piece of parchment paper and store in the refrigerator for about a month.

All-Purpose Nettle Seed Salt

Nettle is a fabulous energy and stamina adaptogen. It's also prolific, easy to grow almost everywhere, and can be used as a green vegetable. Not bad for a hardy little plant that can't quite decide whether to be feral or tame.

Although nettle is an herb that many of us include in our gardens, it will also self-sow freely in semi-tame places such as fields and pastures. Nettle's ambivalence is evident in the trait that gives it its common name, stinging nettle. This plant is quick to remind us with the sharp sting of its feral ways that it wants to be respected for all that it offers. The sting quickly disappears once the herb is cooked or wilted, but nettle should be harvested with long sleeves and gloves, unless you enjoy feeling like you brushed up against an angry horde of ants. I won't judge.

Nettle seeds make for an easy ingredient in seasoning blends. They have a mild taste that is easily disguised as part of the other spices, and they are small enough that you can add them whole. I think they are the perfect condiment for vim and vigor. This recipe is a great all-purpose seasoning blend. If you have some powdered celery seed, feel free to add that too!

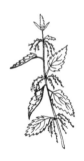

YIELDS 1½ CUPS

½ cup nettle seeds
¼ cup fine sea salt
1 tablespoon powdered
   sage
1 tablespoon powdered
   thyme
1 tablespoon powdered
   parsley
1 teaspoon garlic
   powder

How to Make

1   Nettle seeds are very fine and small, so there's no need to powder them. Mix all the ingredients together in a small bowl.

2   Load some of your new seasoning salt into a salt shaker with a few grains of white rice to absorb moisture. The rice is especially important if you live in a humid part of the country like I do. Otherwise your seasoning blend might turn into a solid block inside your shaker. You can also put your spice blend into a cute salt pig that allows you to give the blend a good poke at every meal with the salt spoon.

3   Store the rest of your blend in an airtight container in the pantry.

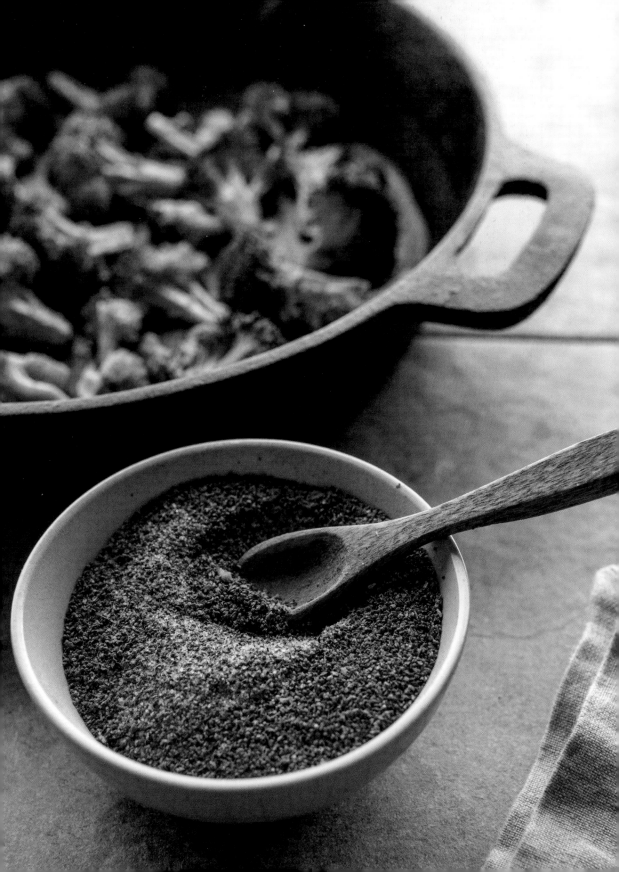

Maca and Suma Maple Syrup

Maca and suma roots are used as foods by native cultures in South America. Here in North America, we tend to treat them as superfoods or potential adaptogens rather than as dietary staples. Both are rich in vitamins, minerals, and amino acids.

It's not necessary to drench your morning pancakes or French toast with this syrup. I use about a tablespoon, and add a little extra plain maple syrup if I want more syrup. The flavor of the two herbs is fairly strong, so it's not as pleasant to take on its own the way an herbal honey can be, but it's still good. Maca has more of a taste than suma in my experience, so you can also try using suma alone if the taste of this recipe is too unusual for you.

Supercharge your morning maple syrup with a decoction of maca and suma!

YIELDS 2 CUPS

½ tablespoon powdered
  maca root
½ tablespoon powdered
  suma root
16 ounces water
1 cup grade B maple
  syrup

How to Make

1 In a medium saucepan with a lid, simmer the maca and suma powders in the 16 ounces of water over low heat for about 20 minutes. The maca will want to stick together in clumps as soon as it hits the water, so you may find that it's easiest to sprinkle it into the water a little at a time. Otherwise you will have to break up a gooey blob of maca powder.

2 Strain the herbs from the liquid and measure to make sure you have 1 cup of decoction. Add a little extra water if needed.

3 Combine the decoction and the maple syrup in the saucepan over low heat. As soon as the maple syrup has dissolved into the liquid, remove the saucepan from the heat. Transfer the syrup to a glass canning jar and store in the refrigerator until needed.

4 To use your maca and suma maple syrup, drizzle about 1 tablespoon into yogurt with fruit, or onto French toast, waffles, or pancakes.

Granola Bites

I love pocket-sized snacks that I can tuck into my backpack or purse, and Granola Bites are delicious and endlessly customizable. Thankfully, gluten-free oats are not nearly as difficult to find (or as expensive!) as they once were, so even if you need a gluten-free option you will most likely be good to go. From what I understand, a small minority of celiacs and gluten-sensitive folks may react to the protein in oats the same way they do to gluten, so check with your doctor if you aren't sure if oats would be right for you.

My mom made my siblings and me a simple peanut butter ball snack when we were kids that consisted of nothing more than peanut butter, powdered milk, and a little honey, so I adopted that trick and almost always add powdered milk to my granola bites for the extra nutrition. You can skip this ingredient if you need to avoid milk.

How to Make

1 Line a baking sheet with parchment paper.

2 Blend together the eleuthero or nettle seed, honey, powdered milk, and nut butter in a large mixing bowl until everything forms a homogeneous paste.

3 Add the oats, cranberries, almonds, and flaxseed or hemp seed to the bowl with the nut butter paste. Knead everything together with clean hands.

4 Divide the mixture into 24 evenly sized dollops on the baking sheet, and roll each dollop between the palms of your hands to create a neat ball.

5 Store the granola bites in the fridge, where they will most likely be good for 2 weeks. If you'd like to make ahead for longer storage, opt for the freezer instead and try to use within a month so they don't get that weird freezer burn taste.

YIELDS 24 BITES (6 SERVINGS)

3 teaspoons eleuthero powder or 6 table-spoons nettle seed
⅓ cup honey
⅓ cup powdered milk (optional)
1 cup nut butter
2 cups rolled oats
1 cup cranberries
1 cup slivered almonds
¼ cup ground flaxseed or hemp seed

Lost in the Wilderness Overnight Steep

Sometimes life feels like a wilderness and you need to keep up your strength. Nettle inhabits our wildernesses, even the very edges of our wild places where we transition from the comfort of home into the less tame. Nettle brings mineral-rich leaves and adaptogenic seeds to this herbal tea.

Elder is another semi-tame herb that haunts our edges of being and wilderness. Myths and legends abound about the elder tree. Most people are familiar with the berries, but not as many know that the flowers have gentle nervine properties. Elderflowers are in this brew for those times when you need to infuse a little myth and magic into your well-being.

Rose hips add a tasty dose of vitamin C and flavonoids, and red clover leaves and blossoms add supportive, nourishing goodness. Both roses and red clover can often be found growing wild. Forage up a batch or buy your supplies from your favorite supplier—whichever you prefer!

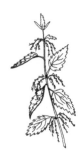

**YIELDS 3 CUPS
TEA BLEND**

1 cup dried nettle leaves
½ cup dried red clover
   leaves and blossoms
½ cup dried elderflowers
1 cup rose hips
2 cups water
⅛ teaspoon nettle seeds

How to Make

1   Blend the nettle leaves, red clover leaves and blossoms, elderflowers, and rose hips together and store them in a labeled airtight container.

2   To make a serving of Lost in the Wilderness Overnight Steep tea, heat 2 cups of water to boiling.

3   Pour the water into a heat-safe glass jar, or leave in the saucepan if you have room to stash it in the refrigerator overnight.

4   Add 2 tablespoons of the tea blend and ⅛ teaspoon of nettle seeds to your brew.

5   Put on the lid and put the container in the refrigerator overnight. In the morning, strain your tea and sweeten it to taste. Sip on your tea throughout the day.

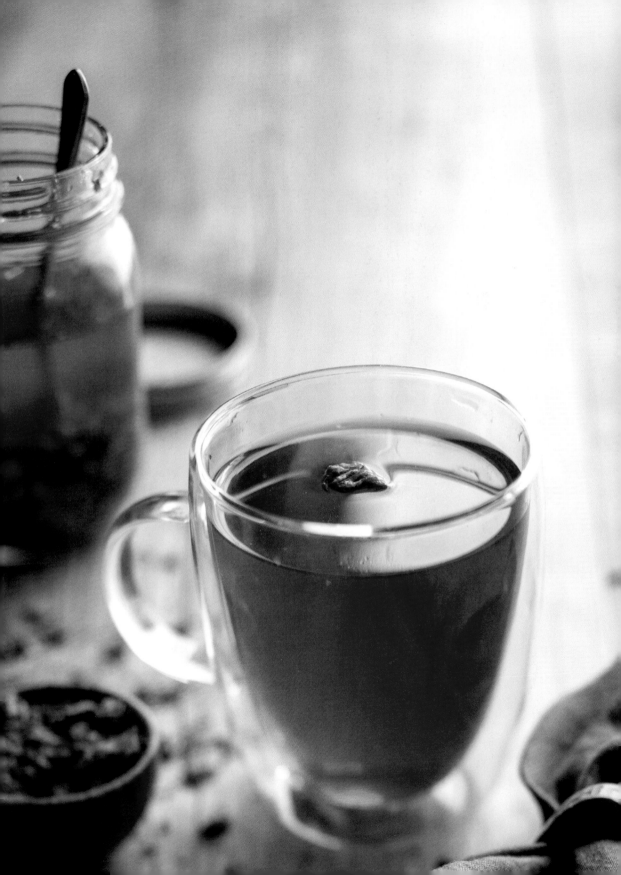

Dang Shen and Hawthorn Blend

Poor man's ginseng, dang shen, forms the base of this formula and teams up with hawthorn for heart and circulation health support and flavonoid-filled goodness. A healthy heart is important for good energy levels, plus both of these herbs provide the usual adaptogenic immune and nervous system support. I add a little coriander to mine mainly for flavor, but it also may have heart-protective nutrients. Feel free to use cinnamon if you don't care for coriander.

Your ability to utilize your nutrients properly also makes a difference in how much energy you have, which is why herbalists sometimes use hawthorn as a tonic for poor digestion. Coriander is a carminative that relieves gas and enhances digestion too.

YIELDS 4 OUNCES

¾ ounce powdered dang shen

¼ ounce powdered hawthorn berries

1 teaspoon powdered coriander seeds

5 ounces vodka or brandy

How to Make

1 Combine the powdered dang shen, powdered hawthorn berries, and powdered coriander seeds in a glass canning jar.

2 Pour in the vodka or brandy.

3 Put a lid on the jar. Store it in a cool, dark place and shake daily for at least 2 weeks.

4 After 2 weeks, strain the mixture, bottle the blend, and label it. Serving size is 30–60 drops and can be taken up to 3 times a day.

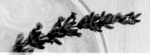

Growing Dang Shen

Dang shen (Codonopsis pilosula) is a hardy, beautiful addition to the garden. It prefers part shade and needs moist soil and regular watering. It's a hardy plant and can handle temperatures down to -15°F. It can even be grown in a container, but it needs a large container rather than a small hanging basket or pot so that the vigorous root system has room to develop. The vine can reach 6 or 7 feet in length and has beautiful small, bell-shaped flowers in the summer, but the stems are fragile. If you decide to try growing it in a container, it may be best to give the plant a permanent home out of the way with a trellis, fence, or pillar nearby so that you don't risk damaging the stems from frequent moving. A trellis is a good idea no matter where you plant it. The roots are sweet and may be as attractive to gophers or other animals as they are to you, so be forewarned that you may need to come to your dang shen's defense!

Coconut Dainties

These dainties are morsels of fantastic nutrition to help you power through your day! I got the idea for these coconut dainties when I was playing around with no-bake truffle recipes and coconut butter. I like how quickly they come together. This recipe calls for coconut butter, which is a little different than coconut oil. Unlike coconut oil, coconut butter contains the dried meat of the coconut, so it has a different texture and a more pronounced coconut flavor.

I love coconut butter for these treats because it suits my "really can't be bothered to bake but want a sweet treat" moods. Do remember that, like nut butter, coconut butter is pretty concentrated stuff, though. A tablespoon of coconut butter (depending on the brand) can have around 90 calories and 18 grams of fat. Compared to almond butter, that's about the same amount of calories but twice as much fat. Some of the fats in coconut are medium chain triglycerides, but most are long chain saturated fats. Depending on which side of the healthy fats party line you like to hang out, you may either scoff at coconut butter as an unhealthy fad, or embrace it as fine in moderation, like most things.

Warm up the coconut butter in a saucepan over low heat for faster mixing, or play around with hand mixing your ingredients. Your hands will warm up the coconut butter after a few minutes, but it's messier than containing everything in a single saucepan. These are best enjoyed cold from the fridge!

Coconut Cranorange Dainties

YIELDS 12 DAINTIES (4 SERVINGS)

6 tablespoons coconut butter
1 tablespoon frozen orange juice concentrate
2 tablespoons chopped dried cranberries (cherries are yummy too!)
1 teaspoon adaptogen powder of your choice

How to Make

1   Melt the coconut butter in a small saucepan over low heat.

2   Add the frozen orange juice concentrate, chopped dried
cranberries, and adaptogen powder. Stir to combine.

3   Pour the mixture into lined miniature muffin tins.

4   These are solid at room temperature, but store best in the
refrigerator.

Coconut Chocolate Hazelnut Dainties

YIELDS 12 DAINTIES (4 SERVINGS)

6 tablespoons coconut butter
2 tablespoons organic or natural brand chocolate hazelnut spread
1 teaspoon adaptogen powder of your choice
2 tablespoons finely chopped walnuts or hazelnuts

How to Make

1   Melt the coconut butter and chocolate hazelnut spread together
in a small saucepan over low heat. As soon as they are melted,
sprinkle in the powdered adaptogen.

2   Add the walnuts or hazelnuts to the mix. Stir to combine.

3   Pour the mixture into lined miniature muffin tins. Once they've
cooled, transfer them to an airtight container for refrigerator
storage.

Coconut, Yogurt, and Fresh Fruit Dainties

YIELDS 12 DAINTIES (4 SERVINGS)

6 tablespoons coconut butter
3 tablespoons plain or vanilla Greek yogurt
3 tablespoons finely chopped berries, apples, or other fresh fruit
1 teaspoon adaptogen powder of your choice

How to Make

1   Warm up the coconut butter in a small saucepan over low heat until it has barely melted.

2   Stir in the yogurt, fresh fruit, and adaptogen powder.

3   Pour the mixture into lined miniature muffin tins and set the tins in the refrigerator to cool. Once they are cold, put them in an airtight container and store in the freezer.

Ginseng Extract

The traditional Appalachian way to preserve ginseng, colloquially referred to as "sang," is to put a fresh root or two into a bottle of corn liquor and allow it to age for a minimum of six months. If you don't have a reputable source for a fresh root, you can still use dried. For dried, I prefer to buy the powdered root as long as I know the turnover of the supplier is high. Powdered herb is exposed to more air, which means faster potential oxidation, but it usually beats trying to grind a whole, dried root by yourself. Coffee grinders don't usually appreciate being enlisted for that task.

Many people don't realize that you can also use ginseng leaves instead of the roots. Some suppliers have started offering this option alongside the roots. It lines up with ethnobotanical usage of the plant, but is still a rare ingredient in modern trade.

There are plenty of choices when it comes to buying your corn liquor. No longer a rare (and illegal) ingredient, these days moonshine has gone legit and has plenty of craft brewing companies providing it for the shelves at your local liquor store. It typically has words like "shine," "white whiskey," or "lightning" in the name.

Give yourself the full benefit of six months of anticipation, or use a percolation method to prepare your extract.

How to Make

1 If you plan to percolate, ready your percolation funnel and the dried ginseng powder, proceeding as outlined in Chapter 1.

2 If you plan to macerate, combine the ginseng powder and the corn liquor in a glass canning jar. Lid and label your concoction, and set it aside for 6 months. Tend it with a good shake every few days and make sure the corn liquor level hasn't decreased thanks to evaporation. If needed, top it off with a little fresh liquor.

YIELDS 3–4 OUNCES

1 ounce dried, powdered
   ginseng root
5 ounces corn liquor

3 After 6 months, filter your extract through a coffee filter to remove the powdered herbs and transfer to an amber glass bottle with a screw cap or dropper top. Make sure you provide your brew with a new label too.

4 Use 60-100 drops up to 3 times a day (roughly ½-1 teaspoon up to 3 times a day).

Super Switchel

Switchel, or haymaker's punch, is a vinegar-based drink that usually includes some combination of molasses or honey, vinegar, and ginger. It's an old-timey drink that originated for summertime refreshment long before sports drinks were invented.

In the summer I like to make a post-run drink that's essentially switchel plus a dash of sodium and potassium from my Super Switchel Salt recipe to replace electrolytes lost from sweating. Super Switchel is an excellent carrier for a serving of rhodiola or eleuthero extract too.

Now for a bit of kitchen chemistry. The typical sports drinks I scouted out on the shelf at the store have around 45mg potassium and 160mg sodium, so that was the same range I wanted for my Super Switchel. Table salt is sodium, of course, but what about potassium? Enter cream of tartar, more formally known as potassium bitartrate. It's usually stocked somewhere in the spice section of the grocery store.

To get 30mg potassium and 143mg sodium, use ½ teaspoon of this blend per 4 servings of switchel, which puts you a tad lower per serving than the sports drinks, but still close. By the way, the bottles I looked at had 2½ servings in each. The first step to make Super Switchel is to blend together a batch of Super Switchel Salt.

Super Switchel Salt

YIELDS ½ CUP (ENOUGH FOR 32 BATCHES OF SUPER SWITCHEL)

¼ cup finely ground salt (sodium)
¼ cup cream of tartar (potassium bitartrate)

How to Make

1 Combine the salt and cream of tartar in a small jar with a tight-fitting lid.

2 Gently shake before each use to make sure ingredients are evenly combined.

Super Switchel

YIELDS 4 SERVINGS

4 tablespoons apple cider vinegar
2 tablespoons honey or molasses
4 cups water
4 tablespoons fresh orange juice
1 tablespoon grated fresh ginger (or more or less, to taste)
4 servings extract of the adaptogen of your choice (either follow the label directions
   or use about 2½ teaspoons of a homemade extract)
½ teaspoon Super Switchel Salt

How to Make

1 Combine all ingredients in a pitcher, place in the refrigerator, and allow to sit overnight for flavors to meld.

2 Enjoy 1 cup post-workout, or pour 2 cups in a water bottle and fill the rest of the way with water for your outdoor adventures.

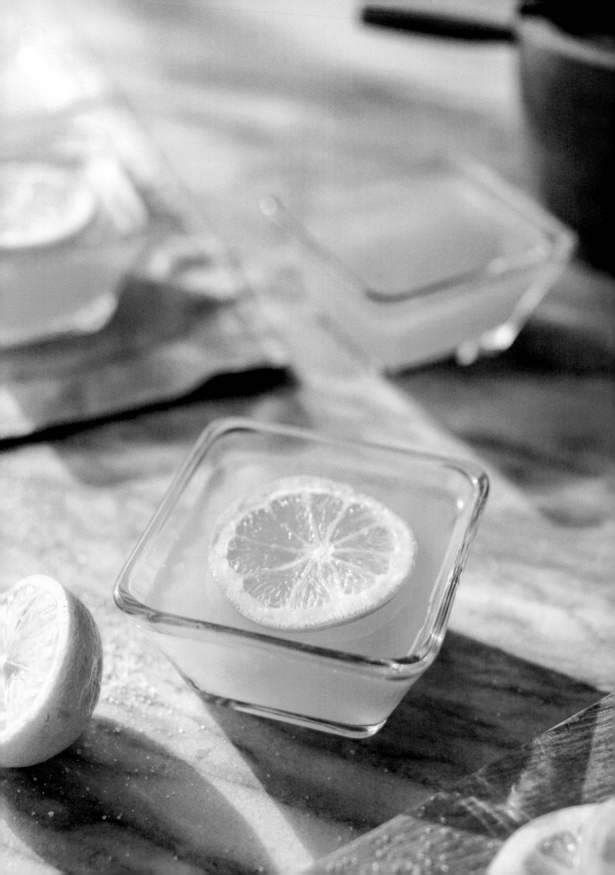

Eleuthero Lemon Gelée

"Gelée" is a fancier word for the jiggly dessert you can find in little boxes in your local grocery store's baking aisle. And this gelatin dessert is special—it has eleuthero in it! A dessert that helps support your energy rather than crashing it from all that sugar? Definitely a go for those on the go! Gelée is a quick make too. It only needs a few minutes of stirring on the stovetop before it's ready to hang out in the fridge.

You can use any juice as a substitute for lemon if you don't like lemon or want to change things up. Make sure to use an equal amount, 2 cups, of your preferred juice if you want to experiment.

How to Make

1   Set out four individual serving dishes. Put them in a small baking pan for easy transportation to the refrigerator in step 5.

2   Pour the 2 cups of lemon juice into a medium saucepan and sprinkle the gelatin over the juice. The juice can be cold or room temperature, it doesn't matter. Allow the gelatin to sit for a few minutes and begin to reconstitute.

3   Heat the juice and gelatin mix over low heat, and add in 3 tablespoons of granulated cane sugar. Stir until the sugar has completely dissolved. Add the eleuthero extract.

4   Pour the juice into the serving dishes, dividing it evenly between the dishes.

5   Move the gelée to the refrigerator and let it set up for a few hours or overnight before you dig in. It will keep for several days as long as you put a piece of plastic film over the gelée or use containers with lids. Garnish each with a fresh lemon slice before serving if desired.

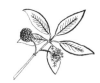

YIELDS 4 SERVINGS

2 cups lemon juice
2 (¼-ounce) packets packaged gelatin powder or 2 tablespoons bulk gelatin powder
3 tablespoons granulated cane sugar
2½ teaspoons eleuthero extract
Fresh lemon slices for garnish (optional)

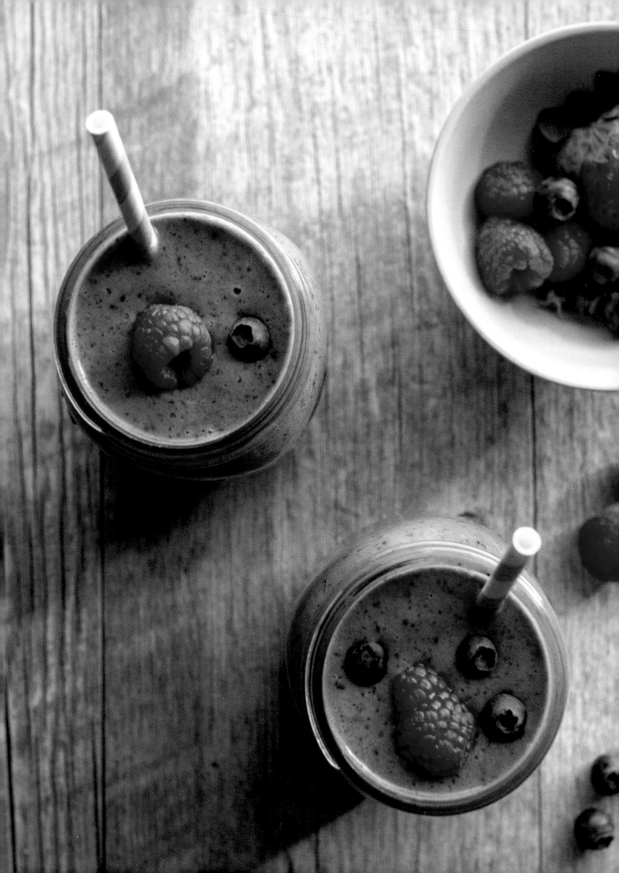

CHAPTER EIGHT

RECIPES TO SUPPORT WOMEN'S HEALTH

Herbs for women can be a complicated topic, but then again, women's health isn't exactly simple, either. Herbs can support us during our major life transitions of menarche, pregnancy, and menopause. They can also help us find balance and comfort during difficult monthly cycles. In each of these cases, though, there's no one-size-fits-all approach. Each woman will experience these stages in her life in different ways, and benefit the most from herbs that are tailored to her unique situation.

Using herbs during pregnancy can be especially tricky. It's best to seek out a qualified herbal practitioner for guidance during such a sensitive time for you and baby, and the use of adaptogens is no exception. There's very little safety information available on the use of adaptogens during pregnancy, and some herbalists feel that it is best not to use this class of herbs during pregnancy. Other herbalists and authors have voiced concerns about the safety of adaptogens during pregnancy based on animal studies or traditions of use, so please don't assume that just because it's herbal and generally safe that the same applies during pregnancy.

Another consideration for herbs and women's health is hormonal birth control. Herbs can potentially alter the way the liver metabolizes things, including birth control pills, or support fertility when you may not appreciate such support. There are not a lot of studies available that look at the ways that herbs can interfere with hormonal birth control, and Saint John's wort is an example of one that seems to be linked to birth control failure. It may also be wise to steer yourself away from herbs like vitex, black cohosh, or even adaptogens that are traditionally used to support fertility. Without studies, there's no way to know for sure, so it's best to talk to your doctor about supplements you want to try if you are on hormonal birth control.

That being said, adaptogens can still be wonderfully supportive for your health and well-being, help you cope with stress, and offer tonic support for women-specific health challenges! Shatavari, in particular, is wonderful for women's health, and so are rhodiola, licorice, and schisandra. Ashwagandha can support a healthy libido, and many of these same herbs offer support during menopause. In this chapter, you'll find recipes for adaptogenic blends, brews, and elixirs that are especially suited for supporting women's health.

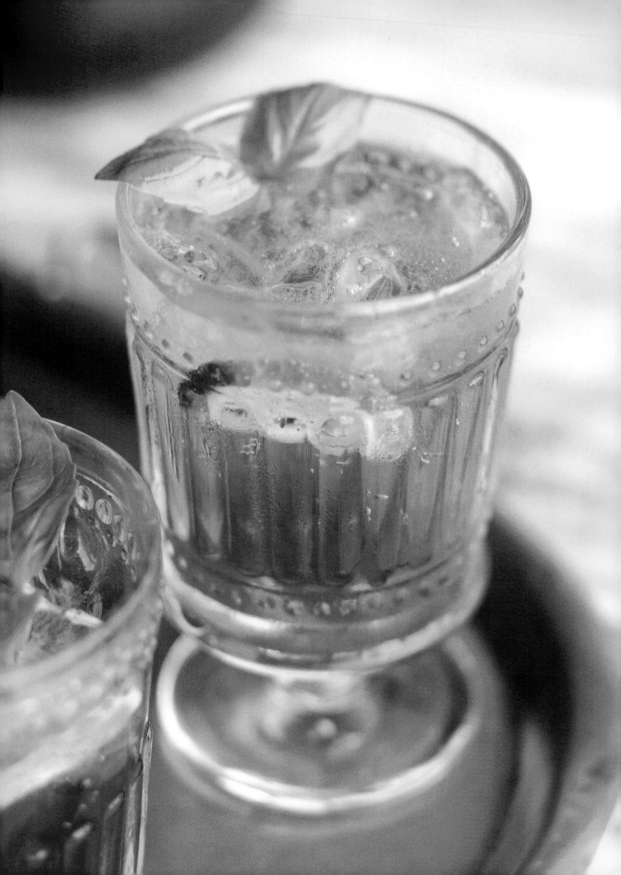

Pomegranate Basil Soda with Rhodiola

Pomegranate juice is a gorgeous dark red color and full of potent antioxidants, so it's a fun treat for adding a boost of extra nutrition to your diet. Pomegranate fruits are usually in season around October, but you can find the bottled juice on the shelf at international markets, health food stores, and some groceries.

Pomegranate is somewhat of a symbol for women's fertility and health, and has had a reputation reaching back into ancient cultures as an aphrodisiac and potent ally for women's health and well-being!

The basil in this recipe is regular garden basil (*Ocimum basilicum*), rather than the adaptogen tulsi (also known as holy basil). They are distantly related, but garden basil is mainly used as a culinary ingredient for flavor, which is its purpose in this recipe too. Using basil along with fruit brings out basil's sweeter side and highlights an almost licorice taste in the herb that is much harder to detect in savory dishes.

Basil grows happily in a container or herb garden as an annual, but you can also often find fresh basil in the produce department of your local grocery store.

How to Make

1 Muddle the basil in the pomegranate juice in a small mixing bowl and then strain out the basil leaves.

2 Mix in the serving of rhodiola extract, and add the seltzer.

3 Add a dash of lime juice, and pour the soda into a glass over ice. Garnish with fresh basil and a lime wedge.

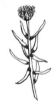

YIELDS 1 SERVING

1 tablespoon fresh basil
½ cup pomegranate juice
1 serving rhodiola extract (follow directions on label or use around ¼–½ teaspoon homemade rhodiola extract)
½ cup seltzer or still water
Dash lime juice
Fresh basil, for garnish
Lime wedge, for garnish

Shatavari Honey and Figs

An electuary is a paste of herbs and honey that can also include dried fruit pieces. In this recipe, the base of the electuary is mostly fig paste with a little honey added for a smooth treat that goes well in yogurt, smoothies, or a glass of almond milk. You can use up to a tablespoon of this electuary at a time.

This electuary contains water that rehydrates the fruit and makes it easier to blend. That means that the electuary may not be as shelf stable as electuaries that don't contain water. Be sure to store Shatavari Honey and Figs in the refrigerator to prevent spoilage. It should store for a month or so. I used Black Mission figs for this recipe but you can use other figs too.

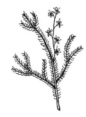

**YIELDS 2 CUPS
(48 (1-TEASPOON)
SERVINGS)**

1 cup chopped dried
Black Mission figs
1 cup water
¼ cup honey
1–2 tablespoons
shatavari powder

How to Make

1   Put the figs into a glass canning jar and allow to soak overnight in 1 cup of water.

2   After they have soaked overnight, transfer the figs and soaking water into a blender or food processor. The figs will most likely have soaked up most of the water, so don't worry if there isn't much water left in the jar.

3   Add the honey and shatavari powder to the figs and water in the blender.

4   Blend the ingredients together until a smooth, paste-like consistency is achieved.

5   Store the finished paste in an airtight container in the refrigerator.

Roseroot Potion

This particular potion helps when that time of the month comes around and you feel a little out of sorts emotionally, and perhaps are struggling physically too. Besides the emotional and physical fatigue that can creep over you, physical setbacks such as cramping and heavy flows can add to the discomfort. Although yarrow is my favorite astringent herb to turn to during this time of the month, there are several adaptogens that can help with the whole shebang.

One of rhodiola's other names is roseroot, and the roots do have a scent that's very similar to rose petals. The compounds in rhodiola that may be responsible for its actions are known as rosavins. Rhodiola has the same ability to bring balance to the endocrine system that all adaptogens possess to some degree. For women's health, rhodiola seems to help with hormonal problems when the main root of the problem lies in stress. Rhodiola has nervine properties, too, so it's a lovely adaptogen to keep in mind for emotional support every month.

White peony is mentioned in Chapter 5 as a nootropic, but it's also a wonderful herbal ally that can make "that" time of the month considerably more comfortable. In TCM it's used for menstrual disorders with a constellation of signs that TCM practitioners describe as blood deficiency, but more generally it's a women's tonic with a reputation for smoothing out imbalances that may express as painful menstruation.

The third ingredient in this blend is schisandra. Sometimes schisandra berries are called "five flavor" berries because they have a very complex taste. Different parts of the berries can be sweet, sour, pungent, salty, and bitter. Try holding a berry in your mouth for a few minutes to soften it and then biting down to release the pungent, bitter flavor of the seeds. It's a very unique experience! Schisandra berries have an anti-inflammatory, astringent, and balancing nature that is very welcome in this blend. The other unique property of schisandra berries, an ability to simultaneously calm and stimulate the central nervous system, makes this especially helpful if you find you have trouble focusing and need a mental energy boost without the extra anxiety too much caffeine can produce.

I used a quickie method for this formula that blends all of the powders together and then puts them through a percolation extract process. Although it's not necessary to do it this way, it is nice to know how to do it just in case you run out at an inopportune time! Because the berry powder seems to swell a bit more than the roots, I find that percolation works best if you pack the cone a little more loosely than normal. You can also blend the formula from single tinctures that were extracted separately as another quick fix alternative to the lengthy maceration process. I've given directions for both.

½ ounce powdered rhodiola root
¼ ounce white peony root powder
¼ ounce powdered schisandra berries
5 ounces 80 proof vodka, plus enough to dampen the herbal powders

How to Make

1   Blend the herbal powders together and moisten with enough vodka to give them the texture of damp sand.

2   Follow the instructions provided in Chapter 1 for making a percolation extract. Pack the cone a little more loosely than normal so that the schisandra berries powder has room to expand. I've found that it expands a bit more than the other two ingredients.

3   Once your extract is finished, bottle and label for later use. A serving size of the extract is 30–60 drops, and can be used up to 3 times a day for everyday use. Use 30 drops (about ¼ teaspoon) up to every hour for a short time, such as during the course of a single day, as needed for extra support.

If you would prefer to make your blend using extracts you mixed up separately, the recipe will look like this:

YIELDS 4 OUNCES

2 ounces rhodiola root extract
1 ounce white peony root extract
1 ounce schisandra berry extract

How to Make

1   Combine the rhodiola, white peony, and schisandra berry extracts in a 4-ounce amber glass bottle.

2   Label and store in a cool, dark cabinet.

What's a Cultivar?

Some herbs—like white peony, chrysanthemum, and echinacea—
are better known as showy garden flowers than as herbs. Their
medicinal history largely forgotten, these plants are now bred by
plant breeders with aesthetics—new colors, showier blossoms,
larger or smaller varieties—or disease- and pest-resistance in mind.
These new varieties are known as cultivars. To know if a plant is a
cultivar, look for an extra name in single quotes at the end of the
botanical designation of the plant. So a cultivar of echinacea might
be *Echinacea purpurea* 'Sundown.' You may wish to check at a specialty plant supplier that carries medicinal plants for a variety that
they recommend using as an herb. Although different varieties, or
cultivars, within a species could potentially be interchangeable,
sometimes the genetic modifications that change the appearance
can change the chemical composition of the plant. The cultivars
available at most garden centers were created strictly for the
sake of appearances or for a specific disease resistance—not with
herbal purposes in mind.

By Your Lady's Leave(s)

There's a very old-fashioned expression, "by your leave," that was a polite way of asking permission, but you most certainly don't need anyone's permission to enjoy this healthy brew of red raspberry leaves and schisandra berries!

The leaves of red raspberry brambles are not really a place where most people would think to look for extra nutrition, but they contain plenty of vitamins and minerals that make them nutritive and perfect for overnight steeps, just like nettles. Red raspberry is a very astringent plant. Pay attention to the first sip, and you may notice that it makes your mouth feel a little drier, which is an interesting sensation from a drink. It's not usually a pronounced feeling and it won't make you any thirstier in the long run, but it does illustrate just how astringent this herb really is!

Because red raspberry is a nutritive herb, the leaves are considered safe for everyday use. I like to prepare mine as an overnight steep to pull out as many minerals as possible, with a few schisandra berries thrown in for extra flavor and adaptogenic goodness.

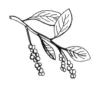

YIELDS 2 SERVINGS

1 quart water
4 tablespoons (¼ cup) dried red raspberry leaves
1 teaspoon dried schisandra berries

How to Make

1   Bring 1 quart of water to a boil and pour into a heat-safe jar.

2   Add dried red raspberry leaves and schisandra berries to the hot water in the jar.

3   Place the lid securely on the jar and allow the berries and raspberry leaves to infuse overnight in the refrigerator.

4   In the morning, strain, and sip throughout the day.

Red Raspberry Leaves

These leaves are a well-loved uterine tonic for women at all stages of life. For teens, they're used to help bring balance to the tumultuous time when we have our first periods. For mothers-to-be, they can nourish our bodies during pregnancy and tone the uterus prior to birth. During transitions to menopause they remain a gently toning, supportive ally for uterine health.

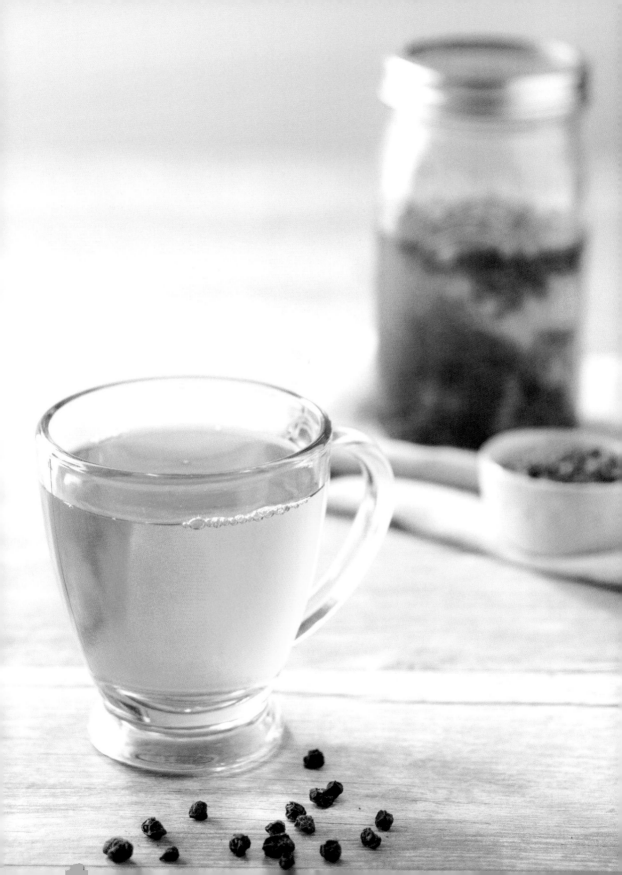

Maca-Choco Truffles

Maca is technically a root vegetable! It's related to radishes, and is a staple of the diet of native cultures that live in the high mountain regions of Peru. It thrives where very few plants can grow, and has a dense nutritional profile despite growing in such inhospitable conditions.

This herb has a reputation for being well suited for endocrine system and energy support, and it always seems to add a little extra pep for me. I admit that I don't really care for the taste of powdered maca by itself, but I have no problem enjoying it in these little coconut truffles!

Maca tends to give me a boost of energy, so I tend to enjoy this recipe early in the day and not as an evening indulgence. I suggest trying it out in the morning or early afternoon as a pick-me-up and seeing how your energy levels respond. Based on your body's response, you can determine how close to bedtime you can comfortably use this recipe.

YIELDS 12 TRUFFLES (4 SERVINGS)

1 cup coconut butter
3 teaspoons maca powder or shatavari powder
3 tablespoons brown rice syrup or agave nectar
1 cup high-quality dark chocolate baking pieces

How to Make

1 Line a small baking pan or tray with parchment paper. This will make cleanup easy, and also give you an easy way to transport your truffles back and forth from the refrigerator while you work.

2 Combine the coconut butter, maca or shatavari powder, and brown rice syrup or agave nectar in a bowl and knead everything together. The kneading may be a little difficult at first, but your hands will warm everything up and it will get easier after a few minutes.

3 Form the coconut butter mixture into twelve small balls and line them up on the baking pan as you work. Place the tray in the refrigerator while you prepare the dark chocolate.

4 Put the dark chocolate pieces into a double boiler over low heat. Stir gently while the chocolate melts.

5 When the chocolate has completely melted, place the tray of coconut balls by your work area and use a spoon to drizzle each truffle with a dark chocolate shell. Once the chocolate has cooled, gently move the balls to drizzle chocolate over the bald spots where the balls touched the parchment paper.

6 Once your Maca-Choco Truffles have cooled, store them in mini-muffin cups in an airtight container in the refrigerator.

Superwoman Shots

Sometimes an extra shot of nutrition is a welcome way to start the day or make it through a mid-afternoon slump. If you own a juicer, feel free to use a shot of your favorite homemade fruit and veggie blend. If you're like me and happen to be sans juicer, you can check in the produce department of your local grocery store for a ready-to-drink greens and juice blend. My local grocery carries several brands and yours might too.

Probiotics are good bacteria that help maintain the health of our digestive systems and can influence everything from our immunity to our mood. The bacteria in our digestive tract actually make up (or should make up) a varied ecosystem with different types of bacteria. We are only just beginning to understand the roles that each kind of bacteria has in supporting the balance of our health. Probiotics were traditionally a part of our diets as fermented and cultured foods like yogurt and lacto-fermented vegetable pickles, but modern diets and an obsession with pasteurization in the name of health and safety mean that our bodies can be missing out on the health benefits associated with good bacteria.

Safely making fermented foods at home is an entire skillset that can bring many fun and unusual foods into our kitchens, but using a probiotic supplement is a user-friendly way to begin adding probiotics back into the diet. In a pinch, you can also open a capsule of probiotics to add to this recipe if you can't find a powdered adult probiotic supplement.

How to Make

1 Pour 1 ounce of greens and juice blend into a small canning jar.

2 Add 1 serving of your favorite adaptogen and 1 serving of probiotic powder blend.

3 Put the lid on the jar and shake everything together. Drink from the jar if you're feeling casual or pour it into your favorite shot glass.

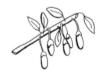

YIELDS 1 SHOT

1 ounce greens and
    juice blend
1 serving adaptogen
    extract of your choice
1 serving probiotic
    powder blend

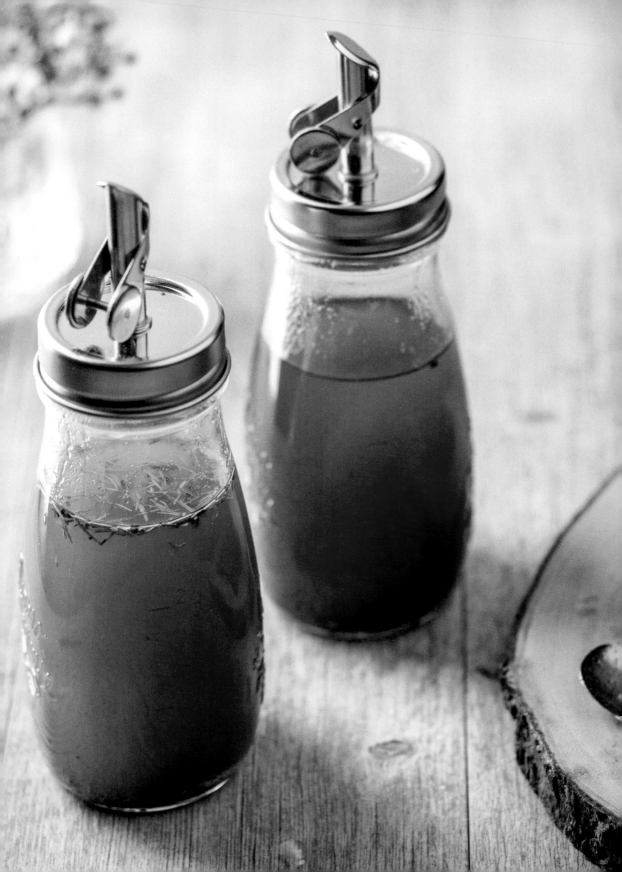

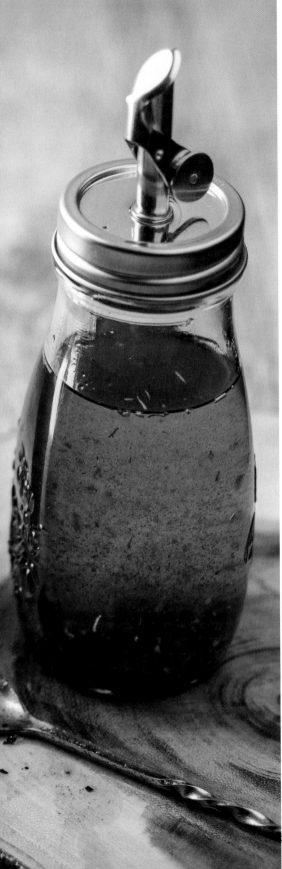

Drop of Magic Kitchen Oils

Don't burn the midnight oil! Instead, add some yummy seasoned cooking oils to your kitchen wizardry repertoire. The extra dash of magic comes from adaptogens, of course!

It's best to used dried ingredients for these oils. Actually, let me rephrase: don't use fresh ingredients for these cooking oils. Fresh ingredients introduce water to the oil, which can lead to spoilage problems and a risk of botulism.

The following recipes include two blends— the Spicy Shatavari Magic and the Herbes de Provence and Ashwagandha Magic—that are easy to incorporate into the kitchen even for less adventurous tastes. The Schisandra and Oregano Oil is a little more unusual, but I think it's still delightful.

The directions I've included call for either combining the ingredients and letting them infuse for two weeks or using a speedy process that includes an overnight double boiler bath in a slow cooker. Choose one of the following recipe blends to get started.

Spicy Shatavari Magic

YIELDS 8 OUNCES

1 tablespoon shatavari powder
2 teaspoons garlic powder
1 tablespoon red pepper flakes
8 ounces olive oil

Herbes de Provence and Ashwagandha Magic

YIELDS 8 OUNCES

1 tablespoon powdered ashwagandha
2 tablespoons herbes de Provence
8 ounces olive oil

Schisandra and Oregano Oil

YIELDS 8 OUNCES

½ tablespoon powdered schisandra berries
1 tablespoon dried basil
½ tablespoon dried oregano
8 ounces olive oil

How to Make via 2-Week Infusion

1 Combine the ingredients for your chosen herb blend along with 8 ounces of olive oil in a glass canning jar and allow to meld for 2 weeks.

2 There's no need to strain the oil; just use as is, a few tablespoons at a time.

How to Make via Slow Cooker

1 Combine the herb blend of your choice and 8 ounces of olive oil in a glass canning jar.

2 Place the glass canning jar into the crock of a slow cooker and add water to the crock. The water should reach halfway up the outside of the glass jar.

3 Turn the slow cooker on to the low setting and put the lid on the glass jar. Leave the lid of the slow cooker on but place a chopstick or similar utensil across the crock and underneath the lid to allow steam to vent. Allow the jar's ingredients to infuse overnight.

4 Turn off the slow cooker the next day and allow the oil to cool before removing it from the slow cooker crock and transferring it to the refrigerator for storage.

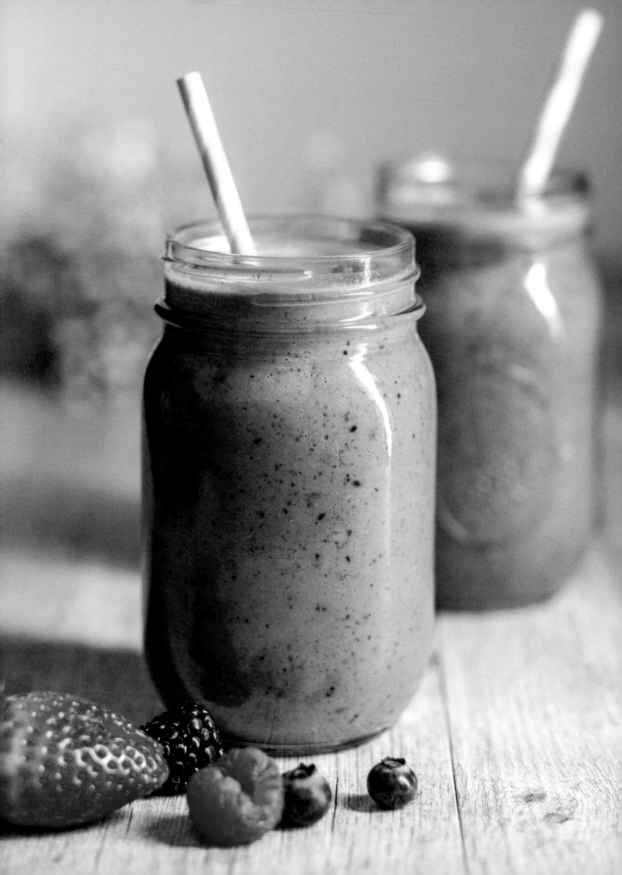

Easy Maca Smoothie

Smoothies are fun nutrition on the go as long as you remember to add plenty of fiber and protein to counteract the sugar rush from all of the fruit! Greek yogurt usually has more protein per serving than other yogurt, and a tablespoon of an all-natural nut butter adds even more. Good sources of fiber include spinach and flaxseed or hemp seeds, but you could also use chia seeds.

I like adding fresh greens to my smoothies. It sounds gross, but you don't taste them in the finished smoothie, and it's much cheaper than adding a scoop of fancy greens powder, although that works, too, if you have it on hand.

How to Make

1   Place the spinach, yogurt, and frozen fruit into your blender and blend them together.

2   Add the flaxseed, nut butter, and maca powder and blend until they have been incorporated.

YIELDS 1 SERVING

3   If your smoothie seems too thick or you have trouble blending all of the ingredients, add a tablespoon of water at a time and try again.

4   Pour your smoothie into a glass, garnish with fresh berries if desired, and serve immediately.

1 cup fresh spinach
½ cup plain or vanilla
    Greek yogurt
1 cup frozen fruit or
    berries of your choice
1 tablespoon flaxseed
1 tablespoon cashew or
    almond butter
1 teaspoon maca powder
Fresh raspberries,
    blackberries, and
    blueberries, for
    garnish

Loving Life Elixir

Damiana and shatavari star as the main ingredients in this recipe. Damiana and shatavari both have reputations as aphrodisiacs, but instead of being an adaptogen, damiana is a nervine that supports the nervous system. The combination of the two is a nice, uplifting blend that works whenever you want a little extra feminine boost—not just in the bedroom!

Shatavari is related to asparagus and also brings some of the same diuretic abilities to the mix. As an adaptogen, shatavari is often used as a gentle nutritive tonic for women's health (although it can be used for men too!), and has a reputation that extends all the way back to ancient times in India. It's even mentioned in the Rig-Veda, a sacred text that dates back to 1500 B.C.E.

Most of the herbal recipes in this book use well-defined measurements, but this is a great recipe for a more relaxed approach that lets you experiment with the folk method of making an extract, which requires no measuring. Use a half pint (8-ounce) canning jar to make a small batch to see what you think!

How to Make

1   Put a thin layer of shatavari root into the bottom of your 8-ounce jar. I usually use about ½ tablespoon. Eyeball it, and use a little more or a little less as the mood suits.

2   Fill the jar about halfway with damiana leaves on top of the shatavari root.

3   Add enough vodka to cover your ingredients by about an inch. You may need to poke the leaves back down into the liquid as you work.

4   Put the lid on the jar and give everything a brisk shaking, then stash the jar in the pantry for up to 6 weeks. Give it a little shake every day and make sure the leaves haven't absorbed all of the vodka. There should be about an inch on top every time you check on it. Add a little more vodka as needed.

5   At any point after 2 weeks, your extract will be ready for use although you can wait as long as 6 weeks before you strain and bottle your extract. When you decide it's time to use your extract, strain out the herbs and pour the extract into a clean glass canning jar. Add in a handful of fresh raspberries and about half the amount of extract in honey. Put the lid on and shake the jar until the honey is combined with the extract.

6   You can begin using your extract at this point or you can wait until it has achieved a level of raspberry flavor that meets your approval. Leave the raspberries in the jar for a few days until you like the flavor, then strain them out and bottle the elixir in a clean amber glass bottle. A serving size is ¼–½ teaspoon up to 3 times per day.

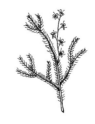

YIELD IS FLEXIBLE/ CAN VARY

Shatavari root
Damiana leaves
80 proof vodka
Raspberries
Honey

Sources for Nettle Seeds

Nettle seeds can be a little difficult to find since most people are interested in the leaves or the roots. Check with your network of local herbalists, add a nettle patch to your own garden, or check through online suppliers of bulk herbs to secure your own supply.

Bee Vital Seasoning

Fennel can be a girl's best friend during times when she needs a little anticramping, anti-bloating goodness with her meal. Parsley, another ingredient in this blend, is a mild diuretic, which can also come in handy.

The nettle seeds provide a vitality boost, while the fennel provides antispasmodic and carminative properties to the mix. Sprinkle this seasoning blend onto grains or use when cooking veggies. Goes well with roasted potatoes too!

The "bee" in this punny recipe name comes from bee balm (*Monarda didyma*; *M. fistulosa*). It's a North American native plant in the mint family with beautiful showy red or purple blossoms. Bee balm has a slightly sweet taste and aroma—almost citrusy—that goes really well with the fennel. If you don't have bee balm (it can be tricky to find unless you are growing your own), use thyme instead. You can use this seasoning blend as a spice while cooking or as a condiment at the table, whichever you prefer.

How to Make

1 Combine the nettle seeds, fennel seeds, powdered thyme or bee balm, and powdered parsley in a small bowl.

2 Store in a cute jar or salt pig on the table where you can easily access it. Use a spoon rather than a spice jar with a sprinkle top so that you can make sure the seeds and powdered herbs stay blended to your liking. Otherwise the heavier fennel seeds will migrate toward the bottom.

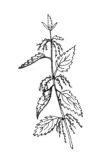

YIELDS ½ CUP

3 tablespoons nettle seeds
3 tablespoons fennel seeds
½ cup powdered thyme or bee balm
2 tablespoons powdered parsley

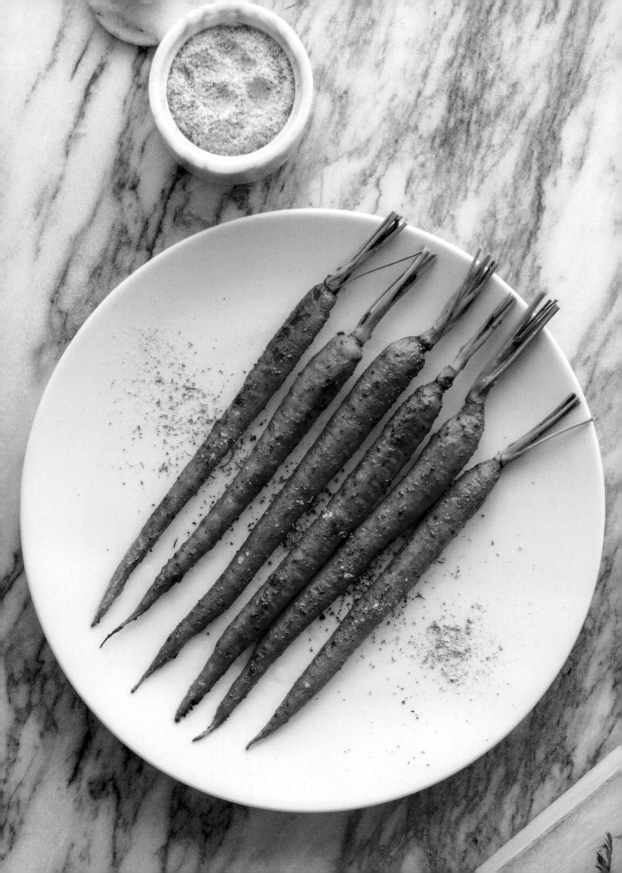

CHAPTER NINE

RECIPES TO SUPPORT MEN'S HEALTH

Besides the ever-popular topics of virility and libido and what herbs can support male reproductive health, prostate health is also an important topic for guys, especially as they reach their forties, and heart health is really important for them as well. There is also room for herbs to support immunity, emotional well-being, and a healthy stress response for the menfolk.

Adaptogens can also offer support in many of these arenas. Ashwagandha, holy basil, jiaogulan, hawthorn, and schisandra are just a few that have nervine properties, support the immune system, and also offer cardiovascular support. Men, say hello to your adaptogenic A-Team.

The recipes in this chapter focus on herbs and adaptogens for overall wellness, heart-healthy spices, and prostate-supporting ingredients, but that's just the beginning when it comes to incorporating adaptogens into a healthy diet for men.

Just, please, guys: don't be tempted to use adaptogens at the expense of your overall health. Adaptogens can support your energy, but that doesn't mean that using them suddenly gives you Marvel comic–style superpowers. Self-care like good nutrition and getting enough sleep may not seem particularly macho, but adaptogens will yield their best results if you are taking good care of yourself!

Superman Shots

A little jolt of extra nutrition and a tasty way to take a serving of adaptogens cross paths in this recipe for Superman Shots. This recipe is modeled on a Bloody Mary. The decision to base these shots on that classic cocktail is not a random one. Tomato juice contains a healthy serving of lycopene, a prostate-healthy antioxidant. Probiotics are important for digestion, immunity, and mood.

If you have fresh tomatoes from a home garden, you can experiment with homemade tomato juice instead of canned tomato juice. I highly recommend trying it if you can, especially with different varieties of heirloom tomatoes so you can enjoy a wider spectrum of flavors in your Superman Shots. The nutrient profile of fresh tomato juice is going to be higher than that of canned tomato juice, too, which is also a plus!

How to Make

1 Combine the tomato juice, Worcestershire sauce, lemon juice, and cayenne in a glass canning jar with the probiotics and your favorite adaptogen.

2 Put the lid on the jar and shake to combine.

3 Drink straight from the jar if you like, or pour into your favorite shot glass.

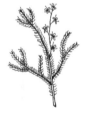

YIELDS 1 SHOT

1 ounce tomato juice
Dash Worcestershire
    sauce
Dash lemon juice
Pinch cayenne pepper
1 serving probiotic
    powder
1 serving adaptogen
    extract of your choice

Pepita Bombs

Pumpkin seeds are a decent source of zinc, a nutrient that has an important job on the prostate health crew. Maca and suma add their dense nutritional profiles to support the endocrine system and energy levels.

In Peru, where it originates, maca is used as a staple food and is one of the few plants that will grow in the harsh environment of the Andes Mountains. It's actually distantly related to radishes, so you might even be able to argue that this recipe counts toward your daily serving of veggies!

Suma is also used for food within its native range, but unlike maca's pronounced, earthy flavor, suma has a mild taste that is a bit like vanilla.

I think these are good with molasses, but if you aren't a fan of molasses you can use honey.

**YIELDS 24 BALLS
(6 SERVINGS)**

½ cup nut or seed butter
1 tablespoon honey or
    molasses
1 teaspoon maca powder
1 teaspoon suma powder
1 cup pumpkin seeds
    (pepitas)
¼ cup shelled sunflower
    seeds

How to Make

1 Mix together the nut butter, honey, maca powder, and suma powder in a medium mixing bowl.

2 Add the pumpkin seeds and sunflower seeds to the bowl and stir everything together.

3 The mix will be easier to work with cold, so let it chill in the refrigerator for about 20 minutes.

4 Once the mixture is chilled, use your hands to roll out 24 small balls. Put them into the container you plan to use for storage as you work.

5 When all of the balls are made, you can store them in an airtight container on the counter or in the pantry. The balls should last a week at room temperature and up to 2 weeks if refrigerated.

Using the Right Amounts

Each recipe is crafted so that one serving of the
recipe gives you one serving of an adaptogen. You
could use up to three recipes per day, or use two
recipes in addition to a plain-Jane serving of extract
or encapsulated herbs. To qualify as an adaptogen
an herb must be nontoxic, but there are still a few of
them that can make you a little uncomfortable if you
get too much. Cordyceps and American ginseng are
probably the two adaptogens that are most important to use at a moderate level.

Cranberry Electuary

Cranberries have a reputation as a fruit for women's health and as a home remedy for urinary tract infections, but they are also really great for guys. They may contribute to healthy high-density lipoprotein (HDL) cholesterol (the "good" cholesterol) levels, and they are a prostate-healthy food too!

Hawthorn and ashwagandha are the starring adaptogens in this recipe. Ashwagandha has endocrine and nervine benefits for men, and hawthorn benefits the cardiovascular system. Hawthorn berries are not a familiar fruit to most people even though they may know about them as an herb. The leaves, flowers, and berries are all used in herbalism, but the berries can also be used to make sauces, jams, jellies, and other preserves, so a little hawthorn berry powder is right at home in this electuary.

Electuaries are usually made with honey and can include fruit. For this one, dried cranberries take center stage for a paste that can be eaten right off the spoon, added to smoothies, or stirred into yogurt.

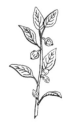

YIELDS 1 CUP

1 cup rough chopped dried cranberries
1 cup water
¼ cup honey
½ tablespoon dried hawthorn berry powder
1½ tablespoons powdered ashwagandha

How to Make

1 Put the cranberries and water into a glass canning jar and let the berries soak overnight.

2 Pour the berries and any leftover water into a blender and blend together.

3 Once the cranberries and water have been blended together, turn off the blender and add the honey, dried hawthorn berry powder, and ashwagandha powder.

4 Blend until all of the ingredients are combined, and transfer to a clean glass canning jar. Use up to a tablespoon at a time. The electuary should keep for about a month, but be sure to store it in the refrigerator.

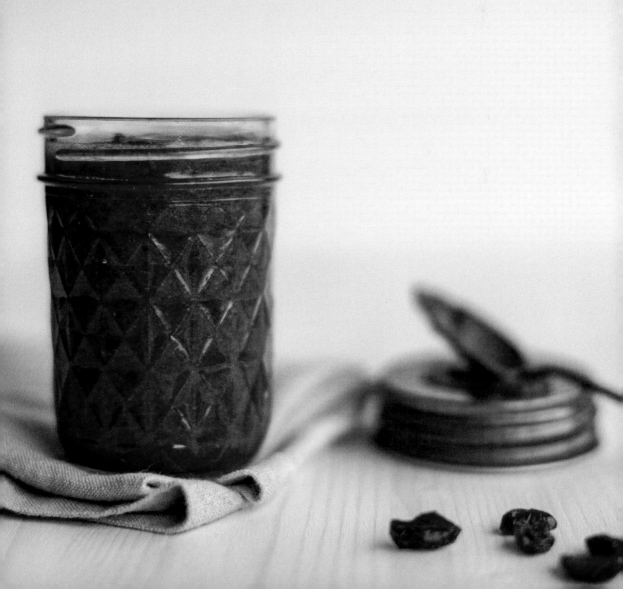

Using Capsules

What if you simply want a quick, easy way to carry a serving of adaptogens with you during the day? Sometimes an extract bottle is a little inconvenient, and you may be wondering whether you can use capsules or tablets of adaptogens. I prefer using teas and extracts because the adaptogens are in a more accessible form; similarly, I like recipes that incorporate adaptogens along with foods because the body is already primed for digestion that way. With a tablet or capsule, your body needs to digest the capsule or tablet and then set to work digesting the plant material in order to get to the compounds in the herbs. As teas and extracts, the herbs have already been "predigested" after a fashion. If you do want to use tablets or capsules, stick with a company that has a reputation for quality across a wide variety of supplements. You can also consider filling your own capsules with a manual capsule-filling machine.

Men's Chai and Mushroom Tea

Because nettle root works best as a decoction, you will want to plan a little ahead to make this recipe. Make the nettle and cordyceps decoction first, and let it brew for 20 minutes. Use the decoction as a base for the chai tea. Choose a loose-leaf chai base that you like for this recipe; I find that a strong black chai is better suited for this than a rooibos.

Nettle root is used in Europe as part of protocols to help the body heal from benign prostatic hyperplasia (BPH), which results from the enlargement of the prostate gland as men age. To be useful for prostate support in that manner, nettle root is best taken daily over several months, or you can use nettle root occasionally as a tonic for the entire urinary tract.

How to Make

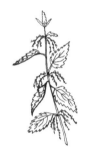

1 Place nettle root and cordyceps in a small saucepan with 16 ounces of water over medium heat. Once the water begins to boil, turn the heat down to low and simmer the herbs for 20 minutes.

2 Strain out the herbs and measure the decoction to make sure there are 8 ounces left. Return the 8 ounces of decoction to the saucepan.

3 Bring the decoction back to a simmer and turn off the heat. Add the loose-leaf chai tea blend or two chai tea bags and place the lid on the saucepan.

4 Allow the chai tea to steep for 5 minutes and then strain the tea or remove the tea bags.

5 Sweeten to taste and enjoy.

YIELDS 1 SERVING

1 teaspoon nettle root
½ teaspoon cordyceps
16 ounces water
½ teaspoon loose-leaf
    chai tea blend or
    2 chai tea bags

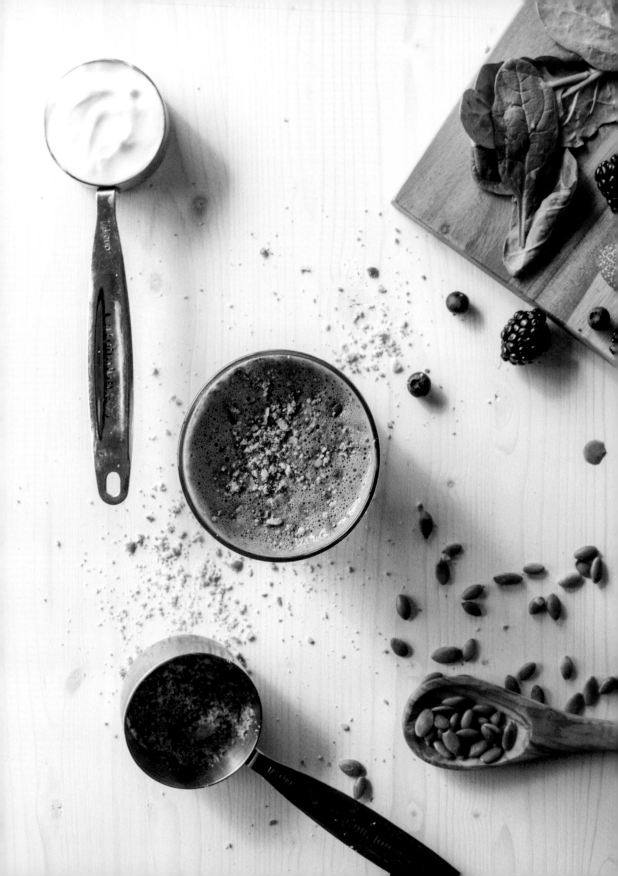

Suma Pepita Smoothie

A pinch of an adaptogen powder in a morning smoothie is a great way to start the day and get some extra nutrition into your daily routine. The fresh spinach may seem like an odd ingredient for a smoothie, but trust me, it's a really good addition and you don't taste it once everything is blended together. You can add a little sweetener of your choice to the smoothie if you like.

With nut butter and Greek yogurt for protein and ground flaxseed for fiber, this smoothie is a great breakfast or afternoon snack. You can experiment with different kinds of frozen fruit to find the flavor that you like the best.

How to Make

1   Begin by putting the yogurt, frozen berries, spinach, and nut butter into a blender. Process everything together until it is nice and creamy. Add a little water if it has trouble coming together.

2   Turn off the blender, and sprinkle the ground flaxseed and suma powder into your smoothie. Put the lid back on the blender and pulse your smoothie a few times to make sure the flax and suma are blended into the mix.

3   Next, you need to make the pumpkin seed topping. Run 1 tablespoon of pepitas through a coffee grinder until you like the texture, or put them in a zip-top bag and roll over them with a rolling pin to crush. You can use a can of soup or similar indestructible item from the pantry if you don't have a rolling pin.

4   Pour your smoothie into a cup and sprinkle the pepita pieces on top.

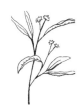

YIELDS 1 SERVING

¼ cup plain Greek
     yogurt
1 cup frozen berries
1 cup spinach
1 tablespoon nut butter
1 tablespoon ground
     flaxseed
½ teaspoon suma
     powder
1 tablespoon pepitas

Man of Legend Truffles

He shou wu has several entertaining myths associated with the supposed power of the roots, including that especially old specimens of the root have the ability to help you grow a new set of teeth or give immortality to the user! Although I love my little he shou wu plant, it doesn't seem particularly magical or likely to do either, but I must say that I haven't had it for such a spectacular length of time.

The raw root does have the superpowers to cause an impressively upset stomach, though, thanks to the presence of anthraquinones. Those are the same irritating ingredients that give senna and cascara (two popular herbs used in bowel cleanse formulas) their laxative properties. Anthraquinones are irritants that can cause dependency if used over time—meaning that if you overuse them you won't be able to move your bowels without them—but it shouldn't be a problem if you're using the processed form of he shou wu. In traditional Chinese herbalism he shou wu is processed by stewing it with black soybeans and then drying it. This makes it much less likely to upset the digestive tract, but it may still have a mild effect on people with very sensitive systems.

He shou wu gets its name, "black-haired Mr. He," from a story about an old man. In the story, Mr. He was very old and ill, but after several years of taking the herb Mr. He's hair turned black again, he was restored to youthful vigor, and he even went on to father children. Considering some of the other tall tales told about he shou wu (immortality? a new set of teeth?), perhaps we should also take this legend with a grain of salt. Still, he shou wu has become a valued herb within several branches of Oriental medicine and is now being studied scientifically as an adaptogen. So we have Mr. He, whoever he may be, to thank for both his personal testimony and some of the wilder, more entertaining conjectures about this plant. Enjoy your Man of Legend Truffles!

How to Make

1. Prepare a baking tray by lining it with parchment paper and set up a double boiler on the stove.

2. Combine the coconut butter, he shou wu powder, and brown rice syrup or agave nectar in a bowl and knead them all together until combined into a paste. The kneading may be a little difficult at first, but as your hands warm the coconut butter it will become easier.

3. Form the coconut butter and herb paste into 12 small balls and set them on the lined tray in the refrigerator while you prepare the dark chocolate.

4. Put the dark chocolate pieces in the double boiler and melt them.

5. Bring the tray of coconut balls back over to your work area and use a spoon to drizzle each truffle with a dark chocolate shell. Once the chocolate has cooled, gently move the balls to drizzle chocolate over the bald spots where the balls touched the parchment paper.

6. Once cooled, store the Man of Legend truffles in mini-muffin cups in an airtight container in the refrigerator. One serving is 3 truffles.

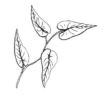

YIELDS 12 TRUFFLES
(4 SERVINGS)

1 cup coconut butter
3 teaspoons he shou wu powder
3 tablespoons brown rice syrup or agave nectar
1 cup high-quality dark baking chocolate pieces

He Shou Wu's Topical Uses

Did you know that he shou wu can also be used topically for skin care? The leaves and vines are sometimes used to soothe itching, and the unprocessed root is applied to unpleasant skin conditions such as boils.

Sarsaparilla and Damiana Potion

Sometimes sarsaparilla is advertised as a men's herb for increasing libido or athletic performance under the same logic used for suma. Herbalists are more likely to note that it is a wonderful alterative. This class of herb gently moves the body into better balance by supporting the channels of elimination. When not being employed as a general whole body tonic, sarsaparilla is traditionally used for things like skin problems, rheumatic disorders, and gout.

Even though it may or may not be a specifically "male" herb, it's still a fine addition to the male herbal arsenal. Plus, sarsaparilla has a distinctive taste that found its way into root beer recipes and makes it a fun extract ingredient. In this recipe sarsaparilla is paired up with a nervine and potential aphrodisiac, damiana.

YIELDS APPROX.
3 OUNCES

½ ounce powdered
   sarsaparilla root
½ ounce powdered
   damiana leaf
5 ounces vodka

How to Make

1   If you like, you can make this recipe with a percolation set up as outlined in Chapter 1. If you'd rather do a maceration extract, follow the instructions here.

2   Place the powdered sarsaparilla root and powdered damiana leaf into a glass canning jar and add the vodka.

3   Put the lid onto the jar and shake it up to soak the herbs in the vodka.

4   Place the jar on a shelf in the pantry and check on it every day for 2 weeks. Make sure there is enough vodka to cover the herbs at all times. If the herbs have absorbed all of the vodka, add a little extra to cover.

5   After 2 weeks, strain and bottle your extract. Make sure to label it. A serving of Sarsaparilla and Damiana Potion is 30–60 drops, and you can use it up to 3 times a day.

Powerblast Popcorn Balls

Besides being popcorn seasonings, adaptogens are the secret ingredient in these easy popcorn ball snacks! You can use adaptogens that have a reputation for being especially suited to men's health, such as suma, maca, eleuthero, or he shou wu, or you can try whatever adaptogen interests you most. It's easy to begin thinking of adaptogens in terms of "his" and "hers," but in reality this isn't a necessary way to categorize them.

Popcorn balls are easy to pack and take along as a snack wherever your busy day takes you, so if you've been looking for portable adaptogen snacking options, try these fun treats.

The pumpkin seeds and sunflower seeds in this recipe are great sources of zinc and protein for immune health and energy levels.

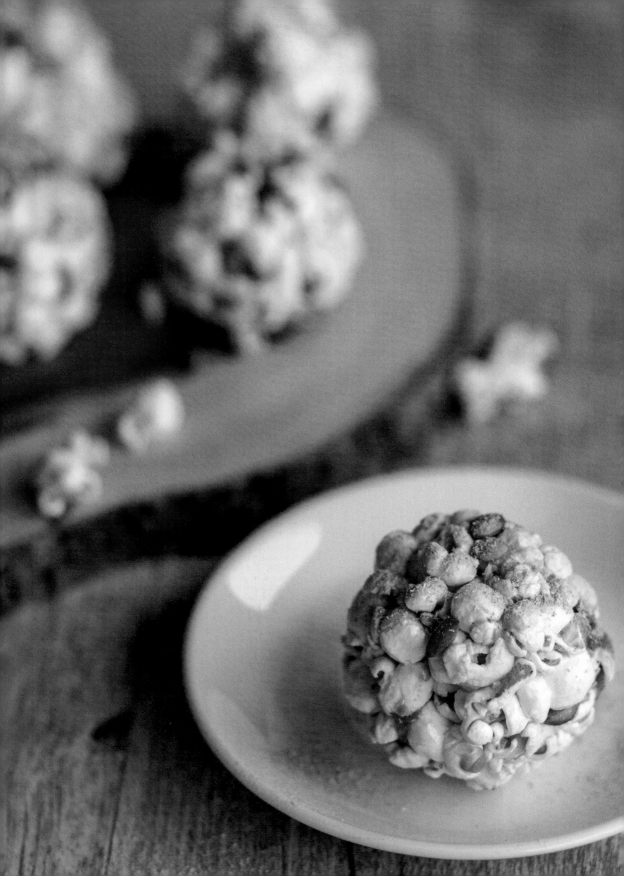

How to Make

1 Line a baking sheet with parchment paper.

2 Melt honey in a small saucepan over low heat. Simmer for a few minutes, giving it a stir every now and then.

3 While it's simmering, measure the popcorn into a big bowl. You want a bowl big enough that you can stir the popcorn around to coat it in the honey.

4 Once the honey has simmered for a few minutes, drizzle it over the popcorn. Stir the popcorn around with your hands to coat it with the honey. Add the pumpkin seeds.

5 You may need to wait 1–2 minutes for the honey to cool before you begin to form the balls. If the honey is too warm it can be a pain to roll the popcorn balls because they are too sticky and won't hold their shape. Form the popcorn and pumpkin seeds into 6 balls of the same size. Line them up on the lined baking sheet as you work.

6 Sprinkle a pinch of your chosen adaptogen onto the top of each ball. Try to divide the adaptogen into even portions on each popcorn ball. If the first batch seems too plain to you, try adding a dash of your favorite spices or seasonings onto the top of each popcorn ball after you add the adaptogens, or stir them into the honey just before you add it to the popcorn balls in step 4 the next time you make them.

7 Store in an airtight container on the counter or in the pantry for 3 to 5 days.

YIELDS 6 POPCORN BALLS (SERVING SIZE 1 POPCORN BALL)

3 tablespoons honey
3 cups plain popped popcorn
¼ cup pumpkin seeds or sunflower seeds
2 teaspoons eleuthero, maca, suma, or he shou wu powder

Powerblast Popcorn Sprinkles

Adaptogens are easily added to popcorn seasoning blends and are disguised well by stronger popcorn seasoning flavors. Flavors that work well as carriers for adaptogens include almost anything spicy or garlic-tinged, ranch, and cheesy blends. Add $\frac{1}{4}$–$\frac{1}{2}$ teaspoon of powdered herbs to a batch of popcorn to sneak in a serving of adaptogens.

Suma Orange Cream Elixir

Suma has a bit of a vanilla taste to it anyway, so playing on that with a little vanilla extract and some orange juice concentrate makes a pretty pleasing elixir blend. Suma's Spanish name is *para todo*, which means "for all things." Pretty big talk for a little root!

You can use a premade suma extract from a reputable company or one that you make yourself. How do you know a reputable supplier for suma? Chances are, the company will offer a full line of herbal products and not just suma. They will also resist making fantastical-sounding claims about suma. If you have doubts about the supplier you are thinking of purchasing from, check the resources guide at the end of this book or pop in at your local health food store (the crunchy one, not the local bodybuilder hangout).

This will ensure that you buy from a company that takes the time to properly identify the ingredients in their supplements, and will also protect you from finding out six months from now that the suma extract you've been using was spiked with something a little extra (and maybe something you would rather not have been putting in your body!). Supplement adulteration scandals do happen from time to time, and the closer you stay to the "crunchy" brands and away from the hype-mongers the better you will protect yourself.

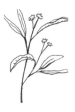

YIELDS 1¼ OUNCES

1 ounce suma extract
2 teaspoons orange
  juice concentrate
5 drops vanilla extract
1 teaspoon maple syrup

How to Make

1   Whisk together the suma extract, orange juice concentrate, vanilla extract, and maple syrup in a small bowl.

2   Bottle and label your elixir.

3   A serving size is 30-60 drops (about ¼-½ teaspoon), and you can enjoy up to 3 servings a day.

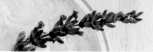

What's the Deal with Suma and Bodybuilders?

Ecdysteroids are compounds found in suma that are important to plant and insect growth processes, and their makeup is similar to that of the human hormone androgen. Suma is thus sometimes marketed as an anabolic agent or as support for healthy male hormone levels because it contains ecdysteroids.

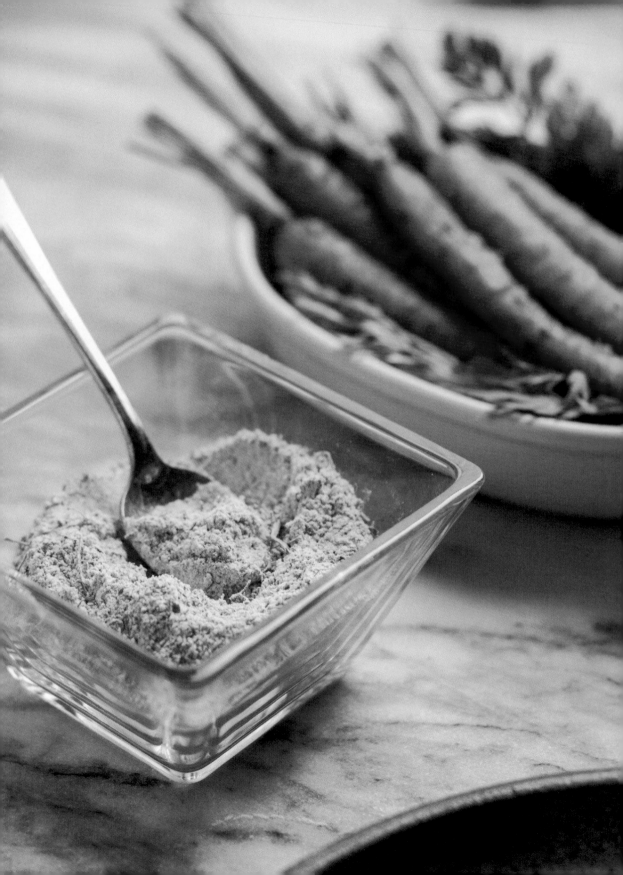

Lionheart Seasoning Blend

Fenugreek and garlic are great spices for heart health. The ancients believed garlic had a fortifying influence when ingested. Roman soldiers would eat garlic before battle to make themselves braver. Or maybe it was just to chase away the enemy with a legion of bad breath.

Garlic has many other uses besides a seasoning in your pantry. In addition to supporting heart health, garlic has been used as an ingredient in cough syrups to help clear the lungs, as an infused oil to fight ear infections, and for sore throats. It's a spicy herb with a fiery personality that can boost circulation to warm up cold hands and feet!

Nettle seeds add some adaptogenic fantastic-ness, and a little parsley in the mix helps keep you from scaring anyone away when you enjoy this tasty blend, since parsley is traditionally used to combat garlic breath.

How to Make

1 In a small bowl, blend together the powdered fenugreek, garlic, cumin, and nettle seeds.

2 Add in the parsley flakes, and transfer the mixture to a small jar. Keep the jar handy on the table so you will remember to add a bit to your plate as a seasoning, or keep it in the spice rack and use it to cook veggies or chicken.

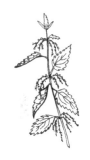

YIELDS APPROX.
¾ CUP
(11 TABLESPOONS)

1 tablespoon powdered
  fenugreek
¼ cup powdered garlic
1 tablespoon powdered
  cumin
¼ cup nettle seeds
1 tablespoon parsley
  flakes

Male Hormonal Health

Even though a man's health isn't as prone to the obvious hormonal cycles that a woman experiences, hormonal balance can still be an important factor for men to explore as they approach their health from a holistic perspective. After around age thirty, testosterone levels in men will naturally begin to decline a little, and some men may begin to experience changes in sleep patterns, mood, and libido due to hormonal changes. Testosterone levels can also be influenced by thyroid problems or other medical conditions, so it's important to be able to discuss hormonal health with your doctor and remember that hormonal health isn't just a women's issue.

Good for the Gander Overnight Steep

Generally speaking, what's good for the goose is also good for the gander. You may think of red raspberry leaf as a woman's herb, but don't be so quick to pass it up. It's a nutritive herb full of vitamins and minerals, and has astringent properties that can support the intestinal tract and urinary tract. Add a little nettle leaf and you have an overnight steep that's great for the gander. So drink up!

You can even add a teaspoon of nettle root to this blend for extra prostate support, but nettle root is generally used on a specific, as-needed basis for prostate health challenges, rather than as a preventive tonic.

How to Make

1 Bring 1 quart of water to a boil and pour it into a heat-safe glass jar.

2 Add 3 tablespoons of dried red raspberry leaves and a tablespoon of dried nettle leaves.

3 Cover the jar. Allow the nettle and raspberry leaves to infuse overnight in the refrigerator.

4 In the morning, strain the leaves out, sweeten the tea to taste, and sip throughout the day.

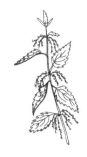

YIELDS 1 SERVING

1 quart water
3 tablespoons dried red
   raspberry leaves
1 tablespoon dried nettle
   leaves

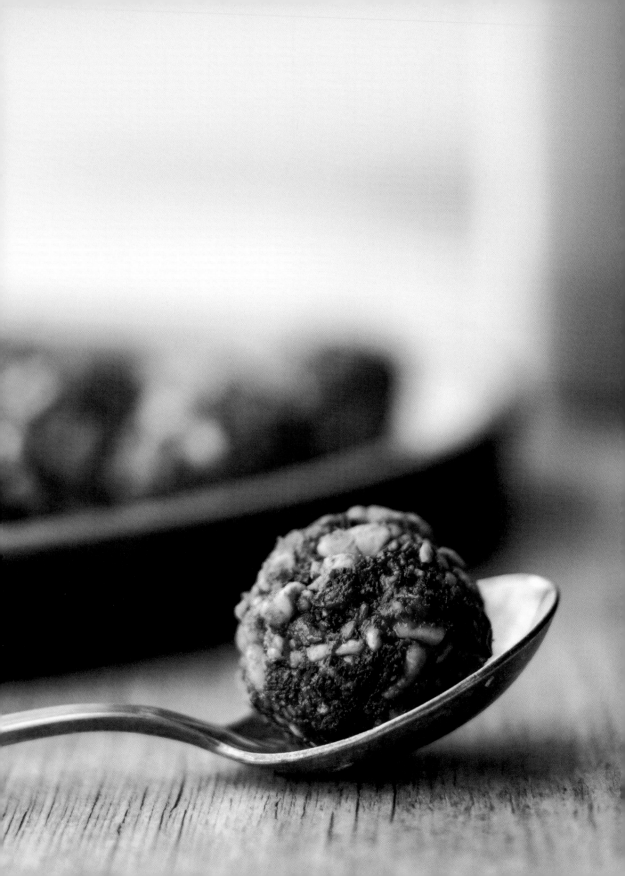

CHAPTER TEN

RECIPES TO IMPROVE YOUR HAIR, SKIN, AND NAILS

In herbalism, we recognize that true beauty comes from the inside out. This is true in the sense that your personality makes a big difference in the way you are viewed by others, but also in the sense that what you put into your mouth for your body to work with makes a big difference!

Beauty superfoods don't have to be exotic. Two of the best things that you can do are eat more fruits and veggies and stay hydrated. Although superfruits like amla and goji get all of the press, most fruits are high in antioxidants. (You should also eat more fiber and cut back on the caffeine.) Some of our best herbal beauty aids are actually a bit on the wild and weedy side and less on the tropical, exotic side. Nettles, oatstraw, red raspberry leaf, and dandelion are full of vitamins and minerals that your body can use for strong, healthy hair, skin, and nails.

Sleep and stress are two other angles to cover with your beauty routine. Make sure that your busy schedule allows you enough time for rest and recuperation! There are plenty of studies that debate whether stress is good for us, or how much is too much, but here's a novel idea: tune in to what your body is telling you about the whole thing.

Once all of your health basics are covered, then you can add some fun adaptogen recipes to your routine. For example:

- He shou wu, in particular, has a reputation for helping your hair's natural beauty really shine through. Amla and goji are full of antioxidants that your body can use for healthy skin.

- In the chapter on nettle in Maud Grieve's *A Modern Herbal*, which was published in 1931, the author mentions that net- tle is an excellent hair tonic and that horse dealers would give nettle seeds mixed in with grain for a few weeks to give their horses a sleek look! So this beauty trick appar- ently works on ponies too.

- Burdock and other gentle alternatives can help cleanse the blood and offer support for any imbalances that manifest in the skin. It's a favorite ingredient in skin clearing brews for many an herbalist, along with herbs such as yellow dock and red clover.

This chapter explores ways to use adaptogens and alteratives for healthy hair, skin, and nails while combining them with light, nourishing foods to supply the body with the building blocks it needs for all-natural beauty.

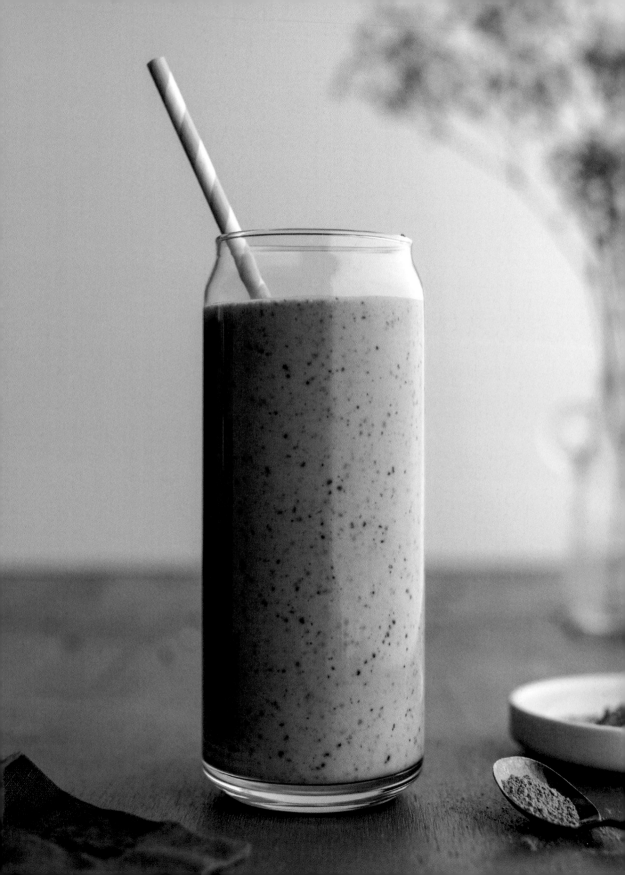

Blueberry Nettle Smoothie

Use a basic nettle overnight steep to infuse extra nutrition into a smoothie already packed with good-for-you Greek yogurt, blueberries, and spinach. A handful of instant oats provides a satisfying amount of fiber. Nettles and spinach are full of vitamins and minerals that pair well with antioxidant-rich blueberries.

To make a nettle overnight steep, also sometimes called a nourishing infusion, you will make a high potency nettle "tea" and allow it to steep overnight so that the maximum amount of nutrients can be extracted from the nettle leaves.

Place 2 tablespoons of dried nettle leaves into a glass canning jar and add 8 ounces of water just off the boil. Place the lid on the jar and allow the nettle to steep for 10–15 minutes, then transfer the jar to the refrigerator. Your overnight steep will be ready to make into a smoothie in the morning! You can add the nettle leaves to the smoothie along with the infusion if you like, or strain them out and use only the liquid.

How to Make

1   Pour the nettle overnight steep into a blender and add the spinach. Blend them together to liquefy the spinach as much as possible.

2   Turn off the blender and add the yogurt, frozen blueberries, and oats and blend some more. Do a quick taste test to determine if you need to add anything to sweeten your smoothie.

3   Pour into a glass and garnish with a sprinkle of matcha powder.

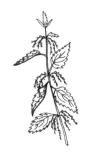

YIELDS 1 SERVING

1 cup nettle overnight steep
¼ cup fresh spinach
1½ cups vanilla Greek yogurt
1 cup frozen blueberries
2 tablespoons instant oats
¼ teaspoon matcha green tea powder

Growing Nettles

I know from experience that this herb does quite well growing in a whiskey barrel-type container. It's not a picky plant. The barrel will limit its size somewhat, but considering that it can reach 6 feet in height and spread in every direction, that's not necessarily a bad thing. Give it rich compost as a potting mix and keep it watered and it will be delighted. If you want to grow it in the ground, be aware that you will easily have a large patch of it in no time if your conditions are right. Nettle grows best in full sun but will adapt to part shade, and prefers rich soil with plenty of water.

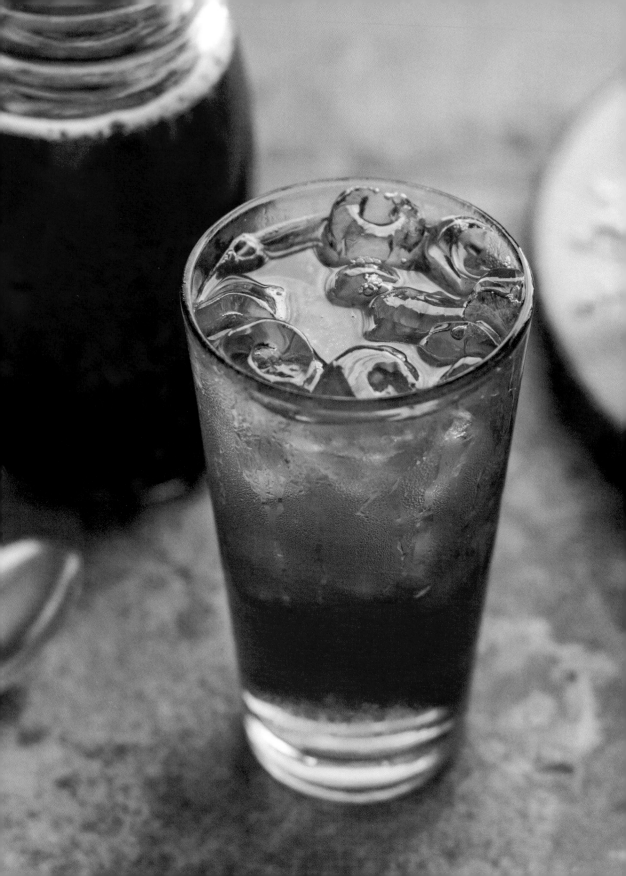

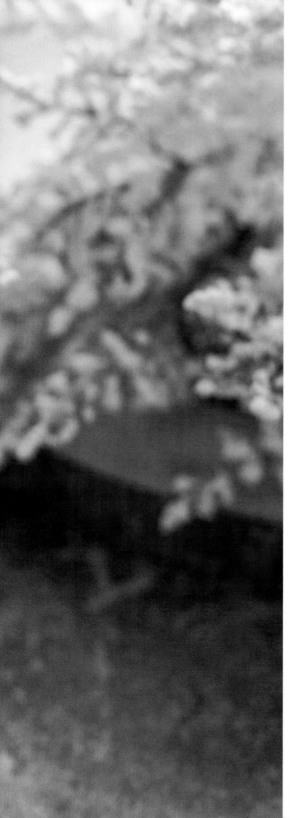

Berry and Blossom Beauty Brew

Antioxidant-rich amla berries team up with red clover for a sippable beauty brew that you can put together at night so that it's ready for you when you're set to start your day.

Red clover is known as an alterative, an herb that helps the body gently detox and eliminate waste, and is used as a tea for clearing and healing the skin from within.

Sugar can trigger an acne outbreak for some people, so you might want to stay away from sweetening your beauty brew. If you really want a sweeter taste for this recipe, I would try sweetening this with a little stevia, which shouldn't cause skin problems.

YIELDS 32 OUNCES
(ENOUGH FOR
1 DAY)

1 tablespoon dried amla
   berries
16 ounces water
24 ounces water
3 tablespoons red clover
   blossoms and leaves

How to Make

1   Simmer the amla berries over low heat for 20 minutes in 16 ounces of water. The decoction will reduce by approximately half, leaving you with around 8 ounces. Transfer the amla berries, and the water they have been decocting in, to a quart-sized glass canning jar.

2   Bring 24 ounces of water to a boil in a kettle. Fill the quart jar with the hot water and add the red clover blossoms and leaves too.

3   Place the lid on the jar and allow it to steep overnight in the refrigerator. Sip on your beauty brew over ice throughout the next day.

Overnight Steeps in the Refrigerator

Some of you might think I'm overly cautious with my recommendation to always let overnight brews infuse in the climate-controlled setting of the refrigerator. Many herbalists are comfortable leaving their infusions out on the counter overnight. I'm not one of them. Even though it's "just" a tea, there's always a possibility of contamination in anything that has come in contact with dirt (hello, plants), or cross-contamination from something on your counters, utensils, or jars. Bacteria has a wild party between about 40°F and 140°F, which, you will note, definitely includes room temperature. While a few hours are probably no big deal, I start getting squeamish about it sitting out any longer than that—like overnight. Refrigerating doesn't hurt the extraction process at all, and if anything, it may enhance it thanks to the movement of the water as it cools. During a cold infusion with herbs such as marshmallow root, we actually rely on the movement of colder water sinking to the bottom of the jar as part of the extraction process. Cold infusion works best if you suspend the herb toward the top of the jar in some cheesecloth, so feel free to play around and let your inner mad scientist have a little fun. But remember to do it at a safe temperature!

Brains and Beauty Bitters

Herbalists will be quick to point out just how important good digestion is for optimum health. One of our favorite tools for keeping digestion in tip-top shape is the humble bitter taste. That's right, "The Taste That No One Likes" is actually really important for health. Just a little taste of bitter primes the entire digestive process from salivation in the mouth on down—all the way down. Yep, even regularity gets a boost from bitters! Bacopa, which is not an adaptogen but is a nootropic (more on those in Chapter 5), is sometimes added to hair and body products for a beautifying boost. It is also known for its pungent, bitter taste.

Dandelion is perhaps one of the most classic examples of an herbal bitter and does a great job keeping the digestive system humming along. Like nettle, dandelion is a very accessible plant because it grows prolifically, much to the chagrin of suburbanites questing after the perfect lawn. Usually the roots of dandelion are used as a bitter, but the blossoms also make an unusual bath and body ingredient for homemade lotions and soaps. I guess that both dandelion and bacopa are "pretty" versatile plants (wink, wink).

All goofiness aside, these two herbs complement each other nicely. There are several ingredients in this recipe to help mellow out the flavor a bit. Will you probably hate it at first? Yes. Is it good for you? Yes. If you keep at it, will you get used to the taste? Possibly. Give it a shot and get your bitter on!

How to Make

1 Combine the dandelion root and bacopa extract in a glass canning jar.

2 Add a pinch of anise seeds, dried orange peel, and a few slices of fresh ginger.

3 Allow to steep together in a cool, dark place for 2 weeks, then strain and bottle your extract.

4 Use a few drops before each meal. Be brave and drop them right in your mouth, or drop them into a little water and knock it back. Remember that the point is to taste them, even if that means diluting them down at first.

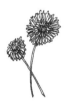

YIELDS 1 OUNCE

½ ounce dandelion root
½ ounce bacopa extract
Pinch anise seeds
Dried orange peel
2–3 (¼") slices peeled
    fresh gingerroot

Beauty Gelée

Gelatin (and its relative, collagen) will periodically get time in the limelight for various health reasons, including promotion as a dietary ingredient to put you on the path toward healthier hair, skin, and nails. In actuality, the body breaks down gelatin and uses the building blocks (amino acids) wherever they're needed, so it's not as though you can absorb it whole and have it go directly to work beautifying. That would be nice, but at least your body is using it for important work.

Gelatin is relatively scarce in the modern diet, but bone broths are one traditional source. A more entertaining way to get some extra gelatin is via dessert!

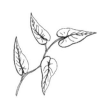

YIELDS 4 SERVINGS

- 2 cups cranberry pomegranate juice (or your favorite berry blend)
- 2 (¼-ounce) packets packaged gelatin powder or 2 tablespoons bulk gelatin powder
- 2½ teaspoons he shou wu extract
- 3 tablespoons granulated cane sugar

How to Make

1   Pour the juice into a small saucepan and sprinkle in the gelatin. Don't turn on the heat just yet. The gelatin needs about 5 minutes to "bloom" and begin absorbing some liquid.

2   After 5 minutes, turn on the stove and heat the juice and gelatin mixture over low heat until all of the gelatin has dissolved. Add the he shou wu extract and the granulated sugar and stir gently until the sugar has dissolved.

3   Pour the mixture into 4 serving dishes and move them to the refrigerator. As the gelatin cools it will begin to set up and take on the jiggle, usually within 4 hours.

4   Once the gelatin is ready, serve your desserts with fresh fruit or enjoy as is!

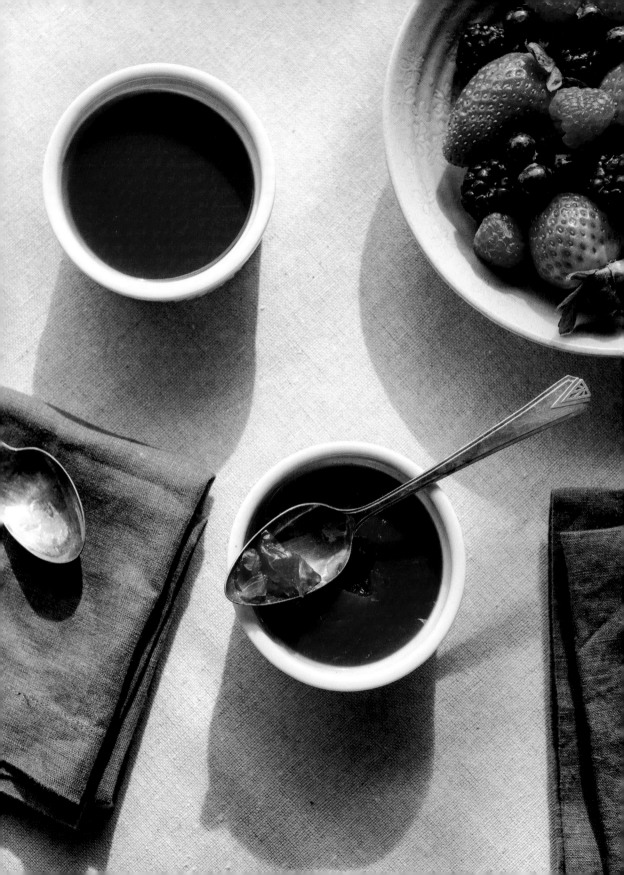

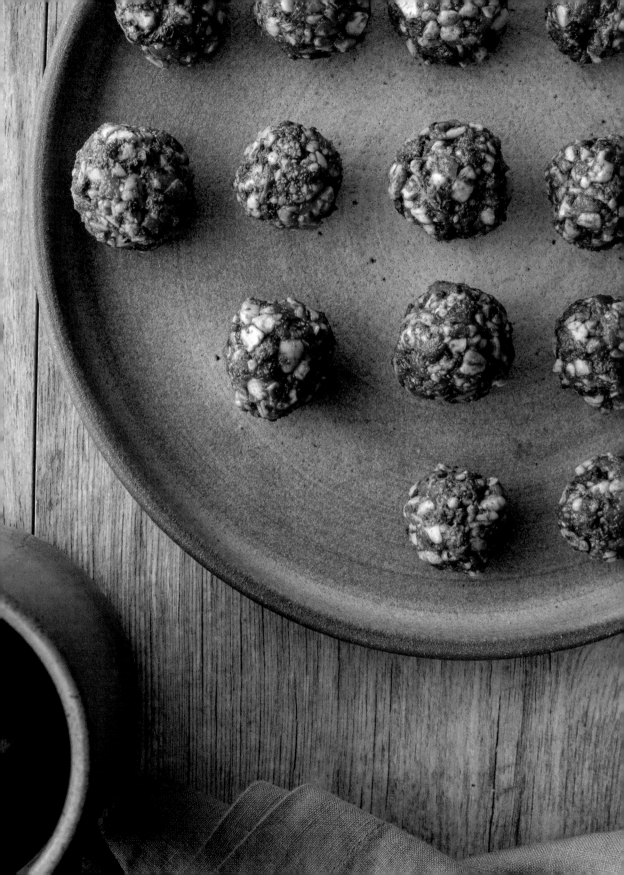

Goji and Amla Bonbons

These tasty little beauty bonbons are made of nothing but fruit and nuts and a little extra sweetener to encourage things to stick together. Goji and amla can help support the health of veins, capillaries, and the skin. Goji also has a reputation for benefiting eye health.

How to Make

1   Let the amla berries rehydrate in a little water overnight. Usually they become very tough and hard when they are dried, but a soak in some water helps to soften them up and make them easier to work with.

2   After the amla berries have had a chance to soften, set them out on a towel and pat them dry to remove any excess water. Put all of the nuts and fruits into a food processor and pulse until everything is in tiny pieces. Be careful not to go too far and let things become a paste!

3   Scoop the nut and fruit mixture into a medium mixing bowl.

4   Drizzle the honey or brown rice syrup over the mixture and use your hands to knead everything together.

5   Using your hands, mold the mixture into little balls once the honey or syrup has been incorporated.

6   Store in an airtight container at room temperature or in the refrigerator. If refrigerated, the bonbons can last up to 2 weeks.

YIELDS 16 BONBONS
(8 SERVINGS)

¼ cup dried amla berries
1 cup nuts of your choice
¼ cup dried goji berries
¼ cup dried apricots
2 tablespoons honey or
    brown rice syrup

Bright Eyes Tea

Goji plus chrysanthemum is a traditional combination, usually with other ingredients such as mulberries, that is used to support eye health. Goji is rich in carotenoids, and we all remember how good the beta carotene in carrots is supposed to be for our eyes. Goji offers comfort for dry, red, watery eyes, and may even be supportive for more serious eye concerns according to traditional use. The same carotenoids and flavonoids that make goji such a sight for sore eyes also make it supportive for fragile capillaries and inflammation that can show up as easy bruising and spider veins.

Chrysanthemum flowers are considered cooling in traditional Chinese herbalism, and also believed to especially influence the liver. The liver and the eyes are linked according to TCM, so their inclusion in the goji and chrysanthemum blends makes sense according to traditional lines of thought. This herb is also considered to be useful for fevers and headaches.

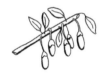

YIELDS 1 CUP

16 ounces water
1–2 amla berries
½ teaspoon goji berries
1–2 chrysanthemum
   flowers

How to Make

1   Bring the water to a boil in a kettle. While the water heats up, drop the amla berries, goji berries, and chrysanthemum flowers into a pint- or quart-sized canning jar.

2   When the water comes to a boil, pour it over the flowers and berries in the jar.

3   Allow your tea to steep for 10 minutes, then strain it into a teacup or mug. Add a little sweetener if desired, but you may find that the goji berries have made your tea sweet enough as is.

4   Discard the chrysanthemum flowers, but you can retain the berries for another cup of tea or two. Be sure to store them in the refrigerator and use them within a few days. Add new chrysanthemum flowers whenever you're ready to make another batch with the berries.

Growing Chrysanthemums

Chrysanthemums are easy to grow as long as you remember a few little quirks of this plant. Mums are perennial, meaning they can come back year after year with a fresh crop of blossoms. Select a variety with white or pale yellow flowers. They need plenty of sun, usually at least 5 hours a day, and mildew can be a problem if the leaves get wet. Mums are great container plants or can be grown out in the garden. When you water them, either set the pot into a tray of water so that the soil in the pot wicks up the moisture or water very carefully underneath the leaves. Watering in a way that wets the leaves and the blooms will cause the blossoms to turn brown and rot (not good if you're planning to make a tea!) and can cause the leaves to mildew. Harvest blossoms when they have just opened and arrange them on a screen in a shady spot or indoors with good airflow so they can dry.

You're probably already familiar with chrysanthemums even though you might not have known their medicinal past. *Chrysanthemum morifolium*, aka "mums," are often sold as garden plants for late summer and fall color. You have probably witnessed their yearly takeover of your local garden center! The varieties most commonly used in TCM had pale yellow or white flowers, but garden enthusiasts go wild for purple, red, and vibrant yellow blossoms.

For this blend, I use amla berries instead of mulberries, but you could try dried mulberries if you have them handy.

Beauty Breakfast Bowl Sprinkle

Goji and he shou wu, plus a little cinnamon, come together for this easy spice blend that goes well on oatmeal or in a yogurt parfait at breakfast time. Up to ¼ teaspoon is 1 serving of this spice blend.

He shou wu is sometimes included in herbal supplements because it is traditionally used when there is premature graying of the hair. In traditional Chinese herbalism he shou wu is classified as a kidney tonic. Although our modern understanding of the kidneys focuses on anatomy and physiological responsibilities, like helping filter waste from our bodies, in the traditional perspective they do much more than that. When viewed from a traditional perspective, the kidneys house the essence of youth and are responsible for overseeing markers of youth, like a clear mind, lustrous hair, and strong bones.

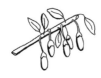

**YIELDS
3 TABLESPOONS**

1 tablespoon powdered
  goji berries
1 tablespoon powdered
  he shou wu
1 tablespoon ground
  cinnamon

How to Make

1 Combine the powdered goji berries, powdered he shou wu, and ground cinnamon in a small glass canning jar.

2 Put the lid on the jar and gently shake the jar to combine all of the ingredients. Let the powder settle to the bottom of the jar before you open it again.

3 Put a few teaspoons of your spice into a salt or pepper shaker, or leave all of it in the jar, whichever you prefer.

4 Apply a label to the jar and store it with the other blends in your spice cabinet.

Legendary Golden Beauty Elixir

Turmeric is the golden party referred to in this recipe's title. *Curcuma longa* is the turmeric we are most familiar with in the West, and is the turmeric called for in this recipe. It has a long tradition of use as a cooking spice. Turmeric contains curcumin, which has been studied for a wide range of health benefits but mainly for antioxidant prowess.

Turmeric provides antioxidants and other compounds for glowing skin from the inside out (or golden skin from the outside in). Don't accidentally drip this anywhere on your face as you're lifting it into your mouth. You might have some temporary turmeric stains on your skin! Turmeric is sometimes used in topical beauty recipes, but considering that it is also used to dye fabric and can impart a yellow tinge to the skin, it might be best to use kasturi turmeric (*Curcuma aromatica*) instead if you want to experiment with topical applications of turmeric.

Internally, turmeric helps provide a healthy dose of curcumin to cool down inflammation and provide protective antioxidants for radiance that comes from within. Being rather bitter, turmeric is more enjoyable as an elixir with honey than as a straight extract.

If you add this extract to water as your preferred method of taking it, you might notice that the turmeric wants to hang out on top of the water. Curcumin isn't water soluble, so that's normal. You can add your Legendary Golden Beauty Elixir to a little sesame oil, milk, or coconut milk instead, which will allow the turmeric to incorporate better and also provide some fats to help with better absorption in the body.

You can use your own homemade extracts for this recipe or opt for store-bought ones.

How to Make

1   Combine the turmeric, burdock, and he shou wu extracts in a glass canning jar and then add the honey.

2   Give everything a few shakes to help the honey dissolve, and then pour the elixir into an amber glass jar.

3   Label your concoction and enjoy. You can use 30–60 drops up to 3 times a day.

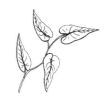

YIELDS 40 SERVINGS

½ ounce turmeric extract
⅓ ounce burdock extract
⅓ ounce he shou wu extract
½ ounce honey

Anointing with Oil for Beauty and Health

Abhyanga is the art of self-massage in Ayurveda. Anointing the whole body with oil is said to have many benefits for health, including boosting skin and muscle tone, promoting better sleep, helping the circulation, and nourishing the body. Abhyanga is believed to be beneficial for all three doshas, but is said to be particularly helpful for the types of people who fall under the vata dosha (doshas are the Ayurvedic descriptions of different body types). Vata people tend to be on the thin side, have dry skin, and have an inquisitive temperament. They may have a lot of nervous energy or spend a lot of time in their heads, so a practice like Abhyanga provides a grounding ritual to help nourish the skin.

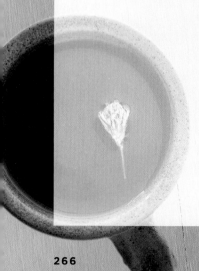

Shatavari Oil

Shatavari roots are usually thought of as a candidate for oral consumption, but they can also be used topically. In folk herbalism, shatavari is infused into an oil and used to treat skin problems. Shatavari also has anti-inflammatory compounds and antispasmodic properties that could lend further benefits to a topical application, whether as part of your facial care routine or as a body oil.

How to Make

1 Place the powdered shatavari root and the sesame or other carrier oil in a pint- or quart-sized glass canning jar.

2 Place the jar into the crock of a slow cooker and add enough water to the crock (not the jar) to come halfway up the outside of the jar.

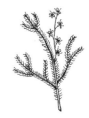

3 Turn the slow cooker to the low heat setting and let the shatavari and oil infuse overnight.

YIELDS APPROX. 8 OUNCES

4 In the morning, turn off the slow cooker and allow the water to cool down to room temperature. You can leave it alone all day if you need to, so don't feel that you must babysit and wait for the oil to cool.

1 ounce powdered
   shatavari root
9 ounces sesame oil or
   other carrier oil of
   your choice
3–5 drops essential oil of
   your choice

5 Once the oil is cool, filter it through a coffee filter to remove the powdered herb. Add 3–5 drops of your favorite essential oil.

6 Bottle your shatavari oil and store in a cool, dark place. If you notice that the smell of the oil changes and turns rancid after a few weeks, discard the oil and make a new batch. You may notice it beginning to smell sharp, musty, or peppery, which signal the oil has gone rancid.

No More Raccoon Root Brew

Too much caffeine can contribute to those dark circles under the eyes as well as fatigue, withdrawal headaches, and other unpleasantness. As we discussed in the Brains and Beauty Bitters recipe earlier in this chapter, bitter dandelion is awesome for digestion, digestion plays a role in the complexion, and burdock helps the body handle its normal detox routines. Here's a bitter black brew for those mornings when you want something coffee-esque—sans the caffeine and plus a little detox boost. Use a plant milk rather than cow's milk for this recipe. The result will be lighter and more appropriate if you are using this as part of a cleanse.

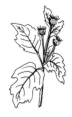

YIELDS 1 SERVING

8 ounces water
½ teaspoon burdock
   root pieces
½ teaspoon roasted
   dandelion root pieces
Plant milk, to taste
Pinch ground cinnamon
   or chai spices
Sweetener of your
   choice

How to Make

1 Bring 8 ounces of water to a boil in a kettle. While you wait, put the burdock and dandelion root pieces into a glass canning jar.

2 When the water boils, pour it over the roots and let them steep for 5 minutes. Strain the roots (you can save them to make another cup).

3 Pour the root brew into a coffee mug and doctor it up with your favorite plant milk, a dash of spice, and a dab of honey, maple syrup, or agave nectar.

Caffeine-Free Energy?

You may hear some people tout the herb guarana as a way to get caffeine-free energy. Unfortunately, this is another "herban" legend. Guaranine isn't responsible for the plant's energizing properties: caffeine is! Not only that, but caffeine is found in pretty high concentrations in the seeds of this South American tree. Coffee weighs in at about 2 percent caffeine by weight. Guarana checks in at up to 5 percent caffeine by weight!

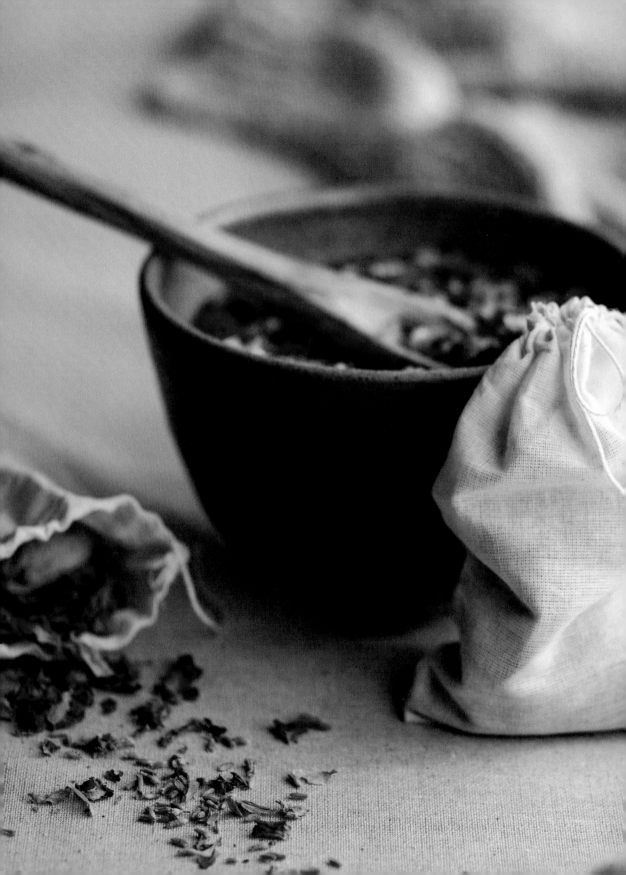

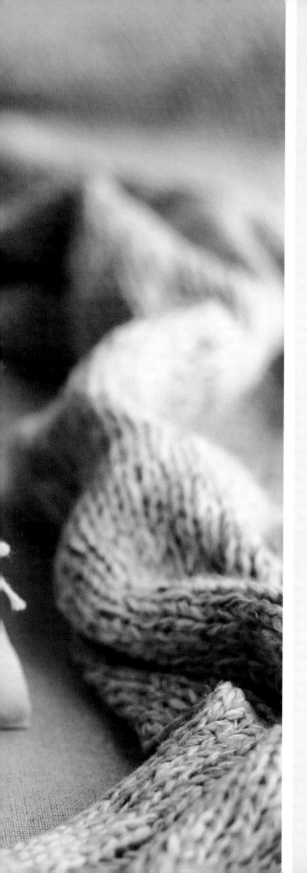

Conclusion: Enjoying Adaptogens Every Day

Hopefully you've been able to see from these recipes that adaptogens can be versatile additions to the diet, and that you can think outside of the capsule or tincture bottle when incorporating them into your health routines. Instead of thinking about a healthy diet as a rigid protocol to be followed, think of it as a series of routines that you can establish that foster a healthy lifestyle. Adaptogens won't replace your body's basic need for a good diet, enough sleep, and good coping skills during stressful times, but they can help support your health through good times as well as bad. Here are a few things to keep in mind as you begin exploring adaptogens and how they fit into your lifestyle.

Adaptogen Don'ts

- Don't rely on adaptogens to fulfill your body's basic needs

- Don't overdo it—too much of a good thing can be a bad thing

- Don't use adaptogens without talking with your doctor if you have a chronic health condition or take prescription medications

- Don't use adaptogens during pregnancy

Adaptogen Dos

- Do incorporate adaptogens into a healthy, balanced lifestyle

- Do enjoy creative ways to add adaptogens to your routines

- Do try different adaptogens and find the ones that resonate the best with your health needs

- Do be mindful that your health needs will change over time and adjust your routines as needed

May your journey to health and balance be a rewarding and creative journey!

Appendix A: Resources and Suppliers

Mountain Rose Herbs

Carries a wide variety of herbs, teas, spices, supplies, tools, and books. Especially to be commended for their dedication to responsible, sustainable sourcing and community outreach to support environmental causes.

www.mountainroseherbs.com

Bulk Herb Store

A good resource for supplies and ingredients.

www.bulkherbstore.com

Strictly Medicinal Seeds

Wonderful selection of medicinal plants and seeds.

www.strictlymedicinalseeds.com

Elk Mountain Herbs

Carries many hard-to-find herbal ingredients, including nettle seeds by the ounce.

www.elkmountainherbs.com

Banyan Botanicals

Focuses on Ayurvedic herbs.

www.banyanbotanicals.com

Starwest Botanicals

A good supplier for all of the basic herbal tools and ingredients.

www.starwest-botanicals.com

Frontier Co-op

Usually this supplier only offers herbs by the pound, but they can be a good back-up supplier or resource if you need large quantities.

www.frontiercoop.com

Gaia Herbs

High-quality extracts and capsules.

www.gaiaherbs.com

Herbs Etc.

Another supplier of high-quality extracts and capsules with some unique formulas.

www.herbsetc.com

Herb Pharm

Excellent resource for many different extracts and compound herbal formulas.

www.herb-pharm.com

Baker Creek Heirloom Seeds

Fantastic supplier of heirloom herb and vegetable seeds.

www.rareseeds.com

Johnny's Selected Seeds

Carries herb seeds as well as vegetable seeds.

www.johnnyseeds.com

LocalHarvest

Connect with herbalists and herb farms with products to sell.

www.localharvest.org

Appendix B: Bibliography

Hoffmann, David, FNIMH, AHG. (2003) *Medical Herbalism*. Rochester, Vermont: Healing Arts Press

McBride, Kami. (2010) *The Herbal Kitchen*. San Francisco: Conari Press

Tierra, Lesley, LAc, Herbalist, AHG. (2003) *Healing with the Herbs of Life*. New York: Crossing Press

Winston, David, and Steven Maimes. (2007) *Adaptogens: Herbs for Strength, Stamina, and Stress Relief*. Rochester, Vermont: Healing Arts Press

Wood, Matthew. (2004) *The Practice of Traditional Western Herbalism*. Berkeley, California: North Atlantic Books

Wood, Matthew. (2008) *The Earthwise Herbal: A Complete Guide to Old World Medicinal Plants*. Berkeley, California: North Atlantic Books

Yance, Donald, CN, MH, RH (AHG). (2013) *Adaptogens in Medical Herbalism*. Rochester, Vermont: Healing Arts Press

US/Metric Conversion Chart

VOLUME CONVERSIONS	
US Volume Measure	**Metric Equivalent**
⅛ teaspoon	0.5 milliliter
¼ teaspoon	1 milliliter
½ teaspoon	2 milliliters
1 teaspoon	5 milliliters
½ tablespoon	7 milliliters
1 tablespoon (3 teaspoons)	15 milliliters
2 tablespoons (1 fluid ounce)	30 milliliters
¼ cup (4 tablespoons)	60 milliliters
⅓ cup	90 milliliters
½ cup (4 fluid ounces)	125 milliliters
⅔ cup	160 milliliters
¾ cup (6 fluid ounces)	180 milliliters
1 cup (16 tablespoons)	250 milliliters
1 pint (2 cups)	500 milliliters
1 quart (4 cups)	1 liter (about)

WEIGHT CONVERSIONS	
US Weight Measure	**Metric Equivalent**
½ ounce	15 grams
1 ounce	30 grams
2 ounces	60 grams
3 ounces	85 grams
¼ pound (4 ounces)	115 grams
½ pound (8 ounces)	225 grams
¾ pound (12 ounces)	340 grams
1 pound (16 ounces)	454 grams

OVEN TEMPERATURE CONVERSIONS

Degrees Fahrenheit	Degrees Celsius
200 degrees F	95 degrees C
250 degrees F	120 degrees C
275 degrees F	135 degrees C
300 degrees F	150 degrees C
325 degrees F	160 degrees C
350 degrees F	180 degrees C
375 degrees F	190 degrees C
400 degrees F	205 degrees C
425 degrees F	220 degrees C
450 degrees F	230 degrees C

BAKING PAN SIZES

American	Metric
8 × 1½ inch round baking pan	20 × 4 cm cake tin
9 × 1½ inch round baking pan	23 × 3.5 cm cake tin
11 × 7 × 1½ inch baking pan	28 × 18 × 4 cm baking tin
13 × 9 × 2 inch baking pan	30 × 20 × 5 cm baking tin
2 quart rectangular baking dish	30 × 20 × 3 cm baking tin
15 × 10 × 2 inch baking pan	30 × 25 × 2 cm baking tin (Swiss roll tin)
9 inch pie plate	22 × 4 or 23 × 4 cm pie plate
7 or 8 inch springform pan	18 or 20 cm springform or loose bottom cake tin
9 × 5 × 3 inch loaf pan	23 × 13 × 7 cm or 2 lb narrow loaf or pate tin
1½ quart casserole	1.5 liter casserole
2 quart casserole	2 liter casserole

Index

About the Author

Agatha Noveille is the founder of the Common Branch Herb School, a grassroots herbal classroom that promotes herbs as a way to safeguard community health and resilience. In addition to writing her own blog, *Indie Herbalist*, Agatha is part of the writing team at the Herbal Academy. She writes regular posts for *The Survival Mom* blog, and has contributed articles to a variety of magazines, websites, and periodicals, including mindbodygreen.com and *From Scratch* magazine. She lives in Dalton, Georgia.